FICTION'S MADNESS

FICTION'S MADNESS

LIAM CLARKE

PCCS BOOKS
Ross-on-Wye

First published in 2009

PCCS BOOKS Ltd
2 Cropper Row
Alton Road
Ross-on-Wye
Herefordshire
HR9 5LA
UK
Tel +44 (0)1989 763 900
www.pccs-books.co.uk

Fiction's Madness

A CIP catalogue record for this book is available from the British Library

ISBN 978 1 906254 23 0

Cover designed in the UK by Old Dog Graphics
Typeset in Times New Roman in the UK by The Old Dog's Missus
Printed by Imprint.Digital.net, Exeter, UK

CONTENTS

Foreword by Femi Oyebode   i

Preface   v

1   What is a Novel?   9

2   Fiction and Madness   19

3   *Regeneration:* Pat Barker   27

4   *Jake's Thing:* Kingsley Amis   39

5   *Richard III:* William Shakespeare   55

6   *The Yellow Wallpaper:* CP Gilman   69

7   *A Most Humourless Solemnity?*   83
     Metamorphosis: Franz Kafka

8   *Felicia's Journey:* William Trevor   101

9   *Macbeth:* William Shakespeare   112

10   *Steppenwolf:* Hermann Hesse   130

11   *Asylum:* Patrick McGrath   145

12   *A Question of Power:* Bessie Head   159

13   *The Good Soldier:* Ford Madox Ford   174

Conclusion   185

Discussion Papers

   1. Chapter 2: *Fiction and Madness*   189

   2. Chapter 12: *A Question of Power*   192

   3. Chapter 7: *Metamorphosis*   195

   4. Chapter 3: *Regeneration*   198

   5. Chapter 3: *Regeneration*   202

   6. Chapter 9: *Macbeth*   205

   7. Chapter 9: *Macbeth*   209

   8. Chapter 10: *Steppenwolf*   212

   9. Chapter 13: *The Good Soldier*   215

   10. Chapter 13: *The Good Soldier*   218

Index   223

For Roman William Wileman,
my beautiful grandson

FOREWORD

In *The Diving-Bell and the Butterfly* (1997), Jean-Dominique Bauby wrote about his experience of 'locked-in syndrome'. This account can be read as a straight account of his experiences, illuminating what it is like for 'a giant invisible diving-bell' to hold one down, like 'a hermit crab dug into his rock'. But, it can also be read as a heroic tragedy; Bauby is the hero who is destined to suffer paralysis but before this travelled, lived life to the full, and without much care. He meets his destiny and in the tragic moment discovers depths of kindness, generosity, and a delight in the sensual and transitory pleasures of life. It can also be read as an allegory for slowness, for stillness, for pensive contemplation in a fast paced, ever-quickening world. Finally, it can be read as a joint creative act between Bauby, his amanuensis and the reader in which the account comes to life in the reading, that is the mind of the reader.

What value can these different readings have for a clinician? Charon et al (1995) have described in what ways literature may be useful to clinical practice: literary accounts of illness can teach concrete and powerful lessons about the lives of sick people; works of fiction about medicine enable clinicians to recognise the power and implications of what they do; understanding about narrative structure can help the clinician to grasp stories of illness more fully; literature can contribute both the texts and methods for a study of narrative ethics; and literary theory itself can offer a healthy counterweight to the dominant mode of understanding of texts and knowledge in biomedicine. These varying insights are as relevant for the clinician in physical medicine as they are for psychologists and psychiatrists. Technical texts have a lot to say about cerebro-vascular accidents in the brainstem but relatively little to say about Bauby's life, the unique qualities and peculiarities of this life and how he would respond to a catastrophe. Yet, out of what, by any description, counts as a shattering irruptive event, Bauby using language in all its magnificence and lyrical beauty, wrought an account that with economy and truthfulness enriches all who care to read it. The manifold possibilities of interpretation give the account openness to traction, a door to the imagination and creative intelligence of the reader.

It is this territory that Liam Clarke traverses in his book, except that his interest is in madness. He takes nine books of fiction and two Shakespearean plays and through these texts explores the nature of madness, with the stated intention of 'promoting better understanding of [madness] above and beyond that provided by textbooks'. He also aims ultimately to work towards 'establishing a more democratic, reflective psychiatry'. This is a book of immense power. It deploys all the devices that literature is capable of to press its case, to argue forcibly and persuasively for the humanising of psychiatry, for an understanding of psychiatric phenomena that goes beyond the rigid borders of descriptive psychopathology. It is a book that demonstrates how fundamental to clinical practice is a familiarity with the humanities, the interpretative and critical domains of our intellectual life. The need for a humane psychiatry cannot be overstated in contemporary life given the new scienticism, the desire for efficiency, for the orderly and sterile, the idolatory of numbers and statistics, the pursuit of spurious precision to the disadvantage of what is properly human and subjective, what grows organically from the complexity and entanglements of human relationships and desires.

I believe that the books that Liam Clarke focuses on highlight his own interests. This is not an attempt at establishing a canon, a prescription of what psychologists or psychiatrists ought to read. Nonetheless the included books are worthy of our interest. Liam Clarke's treatment of these texts is original and enlightening. Borges (1964) in his essay *Kafka and his Precursors* wrote 'I once premeditated making a study of Kafka's precursors. At first I had considered him to be as singular as the phoenix of rhetorical praise; after frequenting his pages a bit, I came to think I could recognise his voice, or his practices, in texts from diverse literatures and periods' (p. 234). Borges is here making the obvious point that reading Kafka sheds light on other writers just as much as these writers also illuminate Kafka. He concludes 'the fact is that every writer *creates* his own precursors. His work modifies our conception of the past, as it will modify the future' (p. 237). Liam Clarke makes links between diverse books, unearths possible interpretations of characters and plots, identifies symbols that cut across culture and gender, and re-fashions our conscious apprehension of particular motifs by awakening in us the unconscious dynamics, the implicit and intuitive communicative aspects of the text. In a word he is modifying our conception of the past and of the future.

Borges (1964) characteristically informs us that 'thinking, analysing, inventing ... are not anomalous acts; they are the normal respiration of the intelligence. To glorify the occasional performance of that function, to hoard ancient and alien thoughts, to recall with incredulous stupor what the *doctor universalis* thought, is to confess to our laziness or our barbarity. Every man should be capable of all ideas and I understand that in the future this will be the case' (p. 70). Borges was preoccupied with the idea that classical texts like the *Quixote* become entertaining books fit only for 'patriotic toasts, grammatical insolence and obscene de luxe editions'. His concern was that fame generated a form of incomprehension, thus a call that we read carefully, analyse and think about what we read. I believe that it is also this desire that partly drives Liam Clarke as he guides and models for us what reading can be like. The act of reading carefully prepares us to listen carefully in the clinical setting, to think and reflect, to consider and engage empathically, and to imagine the world of the Other as if it were our own.

References

Bauby, J-D (1997) *The Diving-Bell and the Butterfly* (Trans, J Leggatt). London: HarperCollins.

Borges, JL (1964) *Labyrinths* (DA Yates & JE Irby, eds). Harmondsworth: Penguin.

Charon, R, Trautmann Banks, J & Connelly, JE, (1995) Literature and medicine: Contributions to clinical practice. *Annals of Internal Medicine*, 599–606.

Femi Oyebode
Professor of Psychiatry
College of Clinical and Experimental Medicine
University of Birmingham

PREFACE

O, let me not be mad, not mad, sweet heaven
Keep me in temper. I would not be mad.
   (Shakespeare, *King Lear*, Act I, sc v)

Few would dissent from King Lear's lament that he not venture from sanity: we can all agree on the wish. More troubling is how not to go mad, how to avoid depression, Churchill's 'black dog', or the existential no man's land of schizophrenia that R.D. Laing (1967: 35) called 'the point of nonbeing … the outer reaches of what language can state'. Perhaps if Laing had attended more the Western literary canon he might have trusted the writer's ability to disclaim insightfully on insanity; poets and novelists writing of love as madness or how to escape it or, for some women, historically, madness as a way *into* it, the flight from male malevolence. All of these themes are covered in the chapters which follow.

This book looks at some links between madness and literature with the aim of promoting better understandings of the former, above and beyond that provided by textbooks. But why tell of mental distress through fiction? In an era of evidence based-practice, biotechnology and pharmacology, it's unfashionable territory. Well, literary narratives might augment psychological knowledge and, consistent with current service user involvement, validate the unorthodox against professional ownership of ideas, thus establishing a more democratic, reflective, psychiatry.

Some voices

Karl Jaspers, a foundational theorist in clinical psychiatry, stated:

> Only through the study of poets such as Shakespeare and Goethe, and writers such as Dostoevsky and Balzac, do we … gain a sufficient store of images and symbols … and … exercise the understanding that is necessary. These all decide whether I remain tied to banal simplifications or whether I endeavour to comprehend men in their most complex manifestations. (1963: 314)

Sound advice, and I have included two Shakespearean works. In total, twelve works are examined for how they address psychiatry in general but, as well, from focused dimensions of feminism, politics, multiculturalism or ethnicity. When choosing these texts I followed my intuitive nose. I didn't canvass colleagues or friends and so some will object to my excluding this or that book, others criticising those included. My selection is therefore idiosyncratic, inevitably so. Let's see what others think.

David Goldberg (2001), a social psychiatrist, has identified Turgenev, Stendhal, Tolstoy, Hardy, Mann, and Vidal as crucial to understanding behaviour. That said, he adds, curiously, that although fiction facilitates understanding of human development, such as links between sexuality, illness and other predicaments, it doesn't contribute to the theory of psychiatry itself. I find this distinction odd especially where illness concepts impact directly on how, where, and with whom we learn to grow into adulthood, in effect to become psychological. Nevertheless, says Goldberg, the distinction is essential to psychiatry's medical standing: that is, psychiatry is abstract, objective, and conceptually independent from fiction, philosophy, opinion, morality. So much for social constructivism! That said, the importance of novels on how one *practises* mental health care is conceded. Quoting Joyce Cary's (1942) novel, *To Be a Pilgrim*:

> They didn't ask me any longer about my wishes. And I did not protest. It was something understood ... that I had no right to protest. I had become a dependent member of the family ... (p. 323)

Goldberg (2001: 89) says that this:

> was a book that made a deep impression on me and taught me more about the experience of growing old and gradually behaving in a way that younger people find eccentric than has any textbook or scientific paper.

But there's a sting in this tail. Referring to Nathaniel West's *Miss Lonelyhearts* (1949) – the story of a male 'agony-aunt' who agrees to meet (but then falls in love with) one of his correspondents – Goldberg anticipates heartbreak and tragedy. In this he employs the classic position of the necessity of boundary between client and practitioner. He allows that the story prepared him for the 'almost limitless suffering and distress that exists in the community' but that it also warned him off proffering *himself* within therapy. As a young doctor he had:

> fantasised about taking the patients I was caring for home for the weekend; but I remembered *Miss Lonelyhearts* and medicated my kindness. (p. 90)

So whilst we enrich our own and our patient's lives via excursions into literature where boundary and division melt in the service of art, we are reminded of the complicatedness of psychiatric work, its emotional precariousness. Of course such warnings are no bad thing. They suggest the limits of psychiatry as a disembodied practice: don't engage with clients, fixate the line of separation between the professional and the other. Thus the essential division between medical psychiatry and other therapists in the field, between the *uninvolved* expert and the empathic listener. Yet when Goldberg was asked, 'what book has influenced you most?' he replied, 'The Brothers Karamazov. I read Dostoevsky in my teens and learned much more about disturbed personalities, human emotions and motivations than from any psychiatric text I have ever read since' (p. 112).

Form and content

Rather than adopt a 'notes' approach, breaking things down to themes, characters, symbols etc., I proffer an essay on each of my chosen books. Professor of Psychiatry Femi Oyebode (2009: ix) quotes D.H. Lawrence (1928):

> Here lies the vast importance of the novel, properly handled. It can inform and lead into new places the flow of our consciousness, and it can lead our sympathy away in recoil from things gone dead. Therefore the novel, properly handled, can reveal the secret places of life: for it is in the passionate secret places of life, above all, that the tide of sensitive awareness needs to ebb and flow, cleansing and freshening.

Without desiring to demean the contribution of formal psychology or psychiatry, I believe that Oyebode's more robust embrace of literature is right. Recalling the late Don Bannister's warning that neglecting everyday language in psychological discourse is risky, I want nevertheless to broaden the spaces between therapist and client from *without*, from a literature that may better situate that discourse distant from medical abstraction but formalised within universally applicable fictions of madness.

One last thing

Whilst each chapter provides much information about the text with which it deals, it goes without saying that the novel or play, if not already known to the reader, must be read as a point of departure. Perhaps, making some notes of psychiatric interest along the way, the reader may be tempted to comment positively or otherwise and to that end here is the author's email address: w.f.clarke@bton.ac.uk

References

Cary, J (1942) *To Be a Pilgrim*. London: Michael Joseph.

Goldberg, D (2001) Ten books. *British Journal of Psychiatry, 178*, 88–91.

Jaspers, K (1963) *General Psychopathology*. Manchester: Manchester University Press.

Laing, RD (1967) *The Politics of Experience and the Bird of Paradise*. Harmondsworth: Penguin.

Oyebode, F (ed) (2009) *Mindreadings: Literature and psychiatry*. London: RCPsych Publications.

West, N (1949) *Miss Lonelyhearts*. London: Gray Walls Press.

WHAT IS A NOVEL?

I wanna tell you a *story*
(Max Bygraves)

One cannot be exact about this. But mainly it is a work of prose, a form of story-telling, of make believe, in the service of human enlightenment. We will discover that inside this general definition await many variations of style, content and method. We will also realise that whilst a product of imagination, the novel has for many years yielded innumerable truths about life in all its forms. What are its particular features? Generally, a novel is longer than a poem, well, most poems. Buying a novel, most of us will expect a 'read' of a certain length. However, this may range from longish works like *War and Peace* (Tolstoy, 1957) to ones like *Regeneration* (Chapter 3), roughly a novel's usual length. Or look at *Metamorphosis* (Chapter 7) which is on the short side, *The Yellow Wallpaper* (Chapter 6) more so. A novel's length is no measure of its depth or breadth however, whether in terms of time – *Ulysses* (Joyce, 1992) is a justly famous (and long) novel spanning one day – or the number and complexity of characters. Anthony Burgess's (1972) *A Clockwork Orange*, for instance, is relatively short but with a full assortment of characters of whom some speak an Anglo-Russian slang called Nadsat whilst the rest speak the Queen's English.

Narrative

Narrative is a novel's way of showing 'what happens next' and is normally the job of a single (and primary) narrator or protagonist. That said, matters can be more complicated. In Hesse's *Steppenwolf* (1965, this volume, Chapter 10), for instance, the main protagonist is Harry Haller but the first narrator we meet is the nephew of Haller's landlady, the second a written text handed to Harry by a stranger and the third is Harry himself, who escorts us to the end of the novel. Thus do novelists play fast and loose with their stories, no doubt anticipating that a bit of literary flash will make us stick with their book.

An important point of narrative is its opening line and some of these are famous in their own right, none more so than Kafka's *Metamorphosis* (1933, this volume, Chapter 7): 'As Gregor Samsa awoke one morning from uneasy dreams he found himself transformed into a giant insect.' Take *Moby Dick*'s (Melville, 1851/2007) startling opener: 'Call me Ishmael.' Or Austen's (1813/

1994) *Pride and Prejudice*: 'It is a truth universally acknowledged, that a single man in possession of a good fortune must be in want of a wife.' This opener is extraordinary because no one in the novel says it, it's Jane Austen talking to us directly, or maybe she's assuming we will suss who *would* have said it as we read on. Two other starters I like are: 'This is the saddest story I have ever heard' from *The Good Soldier* (this volume, Chapter 13) (watch out for a variant on this in *Asylum* (1997: 1; this volume, Chapter 11)) and from Tolstoy's *Anna Karenina* (1954: 13): 'Happy families are all alike; every unhappy family is unhappy in its own way.' These opening sentences are not merely clever, neither do they show evidence of having been overly worked. No, what they do is set a tone for what follows, they are miniature overtures.

Finding the plot

Structure is also important to narrative, how events are programmed so as to make them accessible, recognisable, understandable. This entails 'beginnings, middles and ends' and whose most unmistakable exemplar is 'the whodunit', a genre where carefully planted clues draw readers inexorably towards a conclusion where 'what the butler saw' is revealed. Actually, crime novel aficionados will *expect* things to twist and turn in certain ways and be disappointed if they don't. The same holds true for Mills & Boon fans where if a Mr. Darcy (type) doesn't strut into a drawing-room brandishing a riding-crop, inciting breathlessness in the crinoline-clad bosom's of Regency ladies, well: there just isn't any point in reading on.

Some plots are less prosaic. In *Metamorphosis* (this volume, Chapter 7) Kafka delivers a fable of life, death and pitilessness on the back of a barely perceptible plot. This, evidently, is what Kafka does best, conciseness of form and communication.

> That is why his characters do not always have names. This is not from any refusal to write a proper story; it actually derives from a realisation that so much less was necessary to create a story than people thought.
> (Thirwell, 2005: xiii)

No one was as economical with words than Kafka. Eschewing traditional forms he presents an opening line that decrees his novel's climax and as for 'beginnings, middles and ends', these are replaced with small events such as Gregor's three exits from his room. Says Greenberg (1971: 70):

> *The Metamorphosis* produces its form out of itself. The traditional kind of narrative based on the drama of dénouement – on the 'unknotting' of complications and the coming to a conclusion – could not serve Kafka because it is just exactly the absence of ... conclusions that is his subject matter. His

story is about death, but death that is without dénouement, death that is merely a spiritually inconclusive petering out.

So that when Gregor leaves his room, his degenerating faculties are all the more aggravated as he makes contact with his family; they are his points of human engagement but their resentment hastens his end.

The protagonist

We've observed that the protagonist's 'job' is to carry the story forward. This will normally be a human character (or characters) but may just as well be non-human, the obvious case being science fiction. It may even conceivably be both. In *Steppenwolf* (this volume, Chapter 10) Harry Haller is as much an animal consciousness as someone with a history, social status and so on. And in Edwin Abbott's delightful *Flatland* (2006) the protagonist is a mathematical square caught up in a story about straight lines combating disruptive circles not to mention dangerous triangles and the shenanigans of polygons!

As such, the business of the narrative is frequently complicated by the forms and roles of its protagonist(s). For instance, a narrator/protagonist may comment on another protagonist's actions, the two are not synonymous. Nor may a protagonist remain with a novel till its end, he/she may be substituted along the way. With this collection, you could try working out who the principle mouthpiece of each text is and how they impact on its development. For example, in Amis's *Jake's Thing* (this volume, Chapter 4), given who Jake is, could you expect the story to unravel differently?

Realism

From the eighteenth century through to the nineteenth, novels were realist by nature. That is, they were written so as to be accessible and recognisable (to their readers). Classically, the realist novel is Dickensian and even if some of his characters seem 'panto', nevertheless his work remains credible overall, creating worlds which, suspending disbelief, we accept as true. (Peculiarly, when transferred to the screen – especially the two black and white films directed by David Lean (*Great Expectations* and *Oliver Twist*) – they take on a dreamlike quality, the characters seeming larger than life, at times operatic.) By and large, realist novels have beginnings, middles and ends with matters portrayed as real, the world populated with people you might meet in the street. Even in science fiction, 'characters' will bear some semblance to humans, their communication at least vaguely comprehensible.

From the 1950s, however, novels began to move in mysterious ways and it became difficult to pin them down as a distinct literary form. Suddenly 'Multivoiced narratives, unreliable narrators, allegories, genre dodging, satire, and allusiveness'

(Duguid, 2002: 288) become the order of the day. Novels, including some of those featured here, now deviate dramatically from standard models. No longer are they stories of, let's say, moral improvement or the evocation of an historical epoch. Instead, unusual themes are introduced, writers twisting their stories towards allegory, employing philosophical enquiry and, in some cases, analysing their own novel in the act of writing it. This is not to say that traditional narratives were abandoned. Writers like William Golding retained plausible story lines even when the work in question (*Lord of the Flies,* 1957) was a fable of moral anarchy. And with *Lucky Jim* (1953) Kingsley Amis gave us Jim Dixon, a man not only at odds with 'Merrie England' – he is an historian – but with 1950s stuffiness and academic pretentiousness. Amis's book heralded a change of tone not universally favoured by literary critics. Nevertheless, these two novels, despite their irreverence and audacity, succeeded commercially and critically.

But there also emerged decidedly anti-narrative styles with novels careering into states of mind, linear story lines suddenly bewitched, bothered, bewildered, curtailed, *discarded.* Now might a novel present itself in the process of being written, the author informing you of his technique as you read it. No doubt the intention was to: 'raise the question of whether the pre-eminence of story indulged a populist taste for fantasy, and if other means of writing should be employed to bring the book closer to the random unpredictabilies of life' (Bradford (2007: 5). However, in this, matters went from bad to worse. For example, B.S. Johnson's (1969) *The Unfortunates* comprised 27 sets of loosely bound sheaves of paper (they came in a box) intended to be read in any sequence. Accordingly, the 'creative act' was deployed as a matter of reading as well as writing. Even here, though, small concessions were made with the first and last sections named as such by the publishers (much to Johnson's annoyance!).

In the same vein, but more subtly, some novelists began to embellish narrative with points of theory *about* narrative. Or, they inserted *themselves* into their novel, witness Italo Calvino's *If on a Winter's Night a Traveller* (1981) which starts by informing the reader that he is about to start reading Mr Calvino's new novel! Mr Calvino then proffers advice on how to relax, reminding the reader to turn off all distractions, radios etc. Waugh (2005: 73) mentions a novelist who arbitrarily drops a character in order to make an: 'ontological point about the status of fictional characters as linguistic constructions' and another where a 'missing person' in the story line is not allowed to be found (by the novelist) who instead interjects: 'if he's traced, found, then it all crumbles again. He's back in the story being written'. Confused? You're not alone. This is novel writing that comes from the merger of the theory (of the novel) with actually writing one. It's a combination that's not without its critics. The late Kingsley Amis worked up such a rage against this kind of writing that he swore he'd never read another book that didn't begin: 'A shot rang out!'

Yet for all this, realist novels persist, their characters still required to be psychologically plausible, to be credible. Probably, their creditability has something to do with popularity which demands recognisable forms. Compared to poetry or the theatre, reading novels is phenomenally widespread with thousands published annually. Even 'the telly' has succumbed, witness *Richard and Judy's Book Club* and its yearly selection of 'The Ten Top Books'. So popularity defines (somewhat) what counts as a novel and if some of today's versions seem self-absorbed or unworldly they nevertheless continue as recognisable literary forms.

> What [the novel] reflects most importantly is not the world, but the way in which the world comes into being only by our bestowing form and value upon it. The novel on this view is most deeply realistic not because we can almost hear the sausages sizzling in Fagin's den, but because it reveals the truth that all objectivity is at root an interpretation.
> (Eagleton, 2005: 17)

In effect, a novel's realism is not only what it portrays but comes, as well, from *how* matters are perceived and conveyed in written form. So that, paradoxically, the theoretical elitism of novels that deviate – in their narrative forms – from the everyday are every bit as real when they do this. Which is to say, the everyday emerges through the writer's method and the latter, even when deviant, is just so for a reason, that the everyday is transformed in some way or other.

Into the deep

Realism (and popularity) risk questions such as why hasn't Jeffrey Archer won the Nobel Prize for Literature? After all, his books have strong plots and story lines, are extremely readable – well at any rate widely read – possess memorable characters and relate well to their narrative surroundings. (Actually, Archer, a man with a marvellous ear for character and a great eye for dialogue, is known to entertain ideas of Nobel Prize glory (Mantle, 1989)).

Archer's metier, of course, is popularity (in other words, he produces 'potboilers'), a genre written for sales, contrived, obvious, superficial, derivative. Well, yes, you say, but look at the plot line in *Macbeth* (this volume, Chapter 9); it's a bit transparent in places and Shakespeare stole it! True, but irrelevant. It is the complexity of Shakespeare's characterisation that makes the difference, how his language realises depths of emotion of which the plot line is but the skeleton. Archer's writing, alternatively, is clichéd and overwrought, his novels, like most politician's memoirs, heavily edited by others. But, of course, most people hurtling towards planes, boats, trains or pillows won't *want* much more: the potboiler has its place. And were you to ask six 'serious novelists' to pen 'an Archer' they'd likely buckle beneath the strain. That said, there are plenty of 'Archers' around. Julie Burchill is (an unusual) one in that she has over the years somehow convinced herself that she is a serious writer. You could try her *No Exit* (1993), or there's

Jilly Cooper whose *Riders* (1986) sold millions to persons in search of modest titillation and unwilling to chance the indignity of cruising the Internet.

But some popular storytellers are also good writers. They may not win literary prizes since presumably their work has little internal meaning; not enough *significance* attends their output. To take an example: Robert Harris's novels (1992, 2006) are tremendously well written, having everything a good novel should: story line, character, suspense, strong content, memorable finales. What's missing, apparently, are the indefinable elements that invite interpretation, not so much pleasurable story lines as much as informing the reflective life. So, with a 'literary' writer like Ian McEwan, fiction is not just 'a good read', it's a literature of uncertainty wherein random events influence whomever comes their way. So does Henry Perowne, the surgeon protagonist of McEwan's *Saturday* (2005), encounter sudden intrusions into his life, intrusions which don't just further the story but make points about the incidental nature of living. For instance, McEwan's descriptions of surgical explorations of the brain – he observed operations when researching the book – draw attention to a writer's psychological excavations of character and meaning, both activities, surgical and literary, exposing the human psyche at different levels. This begs an ironic question as to the level at which truth lies, how it corresponds to different methods of investigation. By cutting into their brains, McEwan's surgeon preserves the lives of his patients but about whom he knows little. The novel instead tells us about Perowne, who he is and *why* he is, something that surgery could never do.

If McEwan's work *sounds* contrived, it isn't. His narratives work through real time and place, his characters roundly developed, their experiences deftly woven into the action. At the same time, the meanings he attributes to events recognisably resonate in general terms. This is what serious fiction does and, in his case, does well. In a nutshell, the character's story, in its diverse parts, becomes our story, we are changed by it.

Reading into literature

Most writers hate to talk about their work and often ridicule intellectuals who do. Playwright Samuel Beckett, endlessly invited to explain things, would blankly reply: 'I can't explain my plays. Each must find out for himself what is meant' (Ben-Zvi, 1990: x). This is one of fiction's strengths actually, that it speaks to each of us:

> The house of fiction has in short not one window, but millions – a number of possible windows not to be reckoned, rather; every one of which has been pierced, or is still piercable, in its vast front, by the need of the individual vision and by the pressure of the individual vision and by the pressure of the individual will.
>
> (James, 1963: ix)

But this presumes that fiction *will* elicit responses, be they good, neutral or ill. But were we, for example, to respond to Kafka's *Metamorphosis* (this volume, Chapter 7) where the main character, Gregor Samsa, turns into a bug, with a: 'so what?', then there is no answer to that:

> We can take the story apart, we can find out how the bits fit, how one part of the pattern responds to the other; but you have to have in you some cell, some gene, some germ that will vibrate in answer to sensations that you can neither define nor dismiss. *Beauty plus pity* [original italics] – that is the closest we can get to a definition of art.
> (Nabokov, 1982: 251)

Where beauty exists, says Nabokov, so does pity: and why? Because beauty always dies, the world dies with the individual. Gregor wakes up as an insect and, in doing so, dies and we pity him and ourselves, and if we don't, then we don't.

So why *this* book

Literature's take on human behaviour surpasses the descriptions of social and psychological sciences. The assumption here is that mental health students desire more than the kinds of skills acquisition and detached descriptions which the sciences and even humanistic texts provide. Most mental health problems gather life around them problematically and so it will help to engage practitioners with a literature that runs deep, is more conflicted, that courts the inexplicable things that conventional books don't do. The relevance of this reflects current preoccupations with efficacy, a contemporary milieu that celebrates measurement, compartmentalisation and commodification. It might seem that literary insights are woolly, even at odds with health care's much vaunted 'evidence base'. The scientific approach reduces matters to their atomic elements so as to apply interventions that will modify and/or control those elements. Thus, for instance, is obsessive-compulsive disorder (OCD) disassembled into clusters of stimuli-response mechanisms so as to make them susceptible to treatment by cognitive behaviour therapy (CBT). This therapy originated from theories of maladaptive learning whereby people acquire disabling behaviours though noxious stimuli, to which they later add illogical beliefs and fears which reinforce the behaviours. Today, the effectiveness of CBT across a range of mental conditions is vigorously asserted with many awarding it pride of place within mental health provision. But meaning has its place in these matters too, and truth. One can in fact argue (and I do) that what is therapeutically effective, let's say cognitive behaviour therapy, yields little insight into human affairs, whereas that which lacks therapeutic effect, psychoanalysis perhaps, may yet provide insights of inestimable value into human understanding.

In his short paper, *The Nonsense of Effectiveness* (1998) the late Don Bannister stated that psychotherapy continues to be ruled by medical perspectives. In this, he was referring to therapies dependent on models, yardsticks or frameworks for their points of departure. Wishing to respect conversation in its own right, he went on to say: 'If you were asked how effective is conversation you would surely begin by questioning the question. As it stands it is nonsense' (p. 218). Equally, says philosopher Mary Midgley (2001: 11):

> Words such as care, heart, spirit, sense are tools designed for particular kinds of work in the give-and-take of social life. They are not a cheap substitute, an inadequate folk psychology due to be replaced by the proper terms of the learned.

Terms which, in an evidenced-based milieu, produce mental health workers with limited world-views, nervously unwilling to engage with clients in a relational sense per se. Rather is this text's intention to augment a reductionist evidence base with fiction that amplifies therapies which prize client's narratives within reparative work. The narrative approach is as old as medicine itself as even a cursory look at ancient Greek medicine will show. Psychiatry, however, is a relatively new profession, emerging at a point when medicine was veering away from persons, focusing instead on the body's parts (brain included).

Whereas the psychotherapies have sought to retain the patient's narrative intact, these too have often been formulaic and empire building both intellectually and professionally. As I write, government funded programmes, following the Layard Commission (Layard, 2006), are training thousands of therapists – mainly in cognitive behaviour therapy (CBT) – to respond to a range of disorders. These band-aid practitioners will no doubt eliminate the distresses of some people but there is an attendant risk that the manner in which people author themselves, account for things in their own terms, will be missed. Hornstein (2002: 8), for instance, observes how patient's narratives have become: 'a kind of protest literature, like slave narratives, or witness testimonies. They retell the history of psychiatry as a story of patients struggling to escape despair.' As I have said before, if the exchange is between the pharmacological 'side effects' of muscular twitching, dribbling, the inability to sit for more than a minute and a reduction in voice hearing, some may choose the voices.

This is *the* determinate of this text, to impart some stories of mental distress wherein patients are better understood from a literature that explicates the missing dimensions of the orthodox and the turgid. *The Yellow Wallpaper* (this volume, Chapter 6), one of the texts I have chosen, deals with this issue directly, others do so implicitly. Some examine psychiatry against different historical backgrounds or culturally diverse settings. In addition, *how* these stories are told is also important. For instance, in *Regeneration* (this volume, Chapter 3) psychiatric history is interwoven with fictional characters against a backcloth of war impacting on class, gender and medical power. Here, psychiatric distress and human fate are metaphors for destruction, testimony to how individual experiences of war carry universal significance.

One final point: the narrator may be *unreliable*; he is after all, a character too and we have little choice but to rely on his or her truthfulness. This unreliability is taken to daring lengths in *The Good Soldier* (this volume, Chapter 13) where the narrative is non-linear, wandering backwards and forwards against shifting characterisations. It is also deployed interestingly in *Asylum* (this volume, Chapter 11) where psychiatry becomes the handmaiden of deceit. The unreliable narrator is a difficult concept but makes for more interesting reading because it sustains tension and unpredictability. This is because it is strangely tempting to believe the protagonist, forgetting that, as part of the story, he is as likely to be as dishonest as anyone else.

The texts

Any choice will reflect the tastes of the chooser (obviously) but only up to a point. My chosen books have all merited critical acclaim. They are great fiction of the 'it goes without saying' variety or, if it does need saying, then 'brilliant', 'superb', 'outstanding' may be applied. I have arranged the chapters so that they may be read in any order although, occasionally, some chapters make reference to others and this has necessitated some sequencing.

This is not a book of literary criticism; you will need to go elsewhere for that. Rather is its (modest) aim to underpin clinical literature with 'outsider' views about mental illness, to explore how fiction engages our thinking so as to yield some useful insights, or some poor ones, about how madness is experienced as well how it is traditionally represented.

References

Abbott, EA (2006) *Flatland*. Oxford: Oxford University Press. [Original work published 1884]

Amis, K (1953) *Lucky Jim*. London: Victor Gollancz.

Austen, J (1994) *Pride and Prejudice*. Harmondsworth: Penguin. [Original work published 1813]

Bannister, D (1998) The nonsense of effectiveness. *Changes, 16* (3), 218–20.

Barker, P (1992) *Regeneration*. Harmondsworth: Penguin.

Ben-Zvi, L (1990) *Women in Beckett*. Urbana, IL: University of Illinois Press.

Bradford, R (2007) *The Novel Now*. Oxford: Blackwell.

Burchill, J (1993) *No Exit*. London: Sinclair Stevenson.

Burgess, A (1972) *A Clockwork Orange*. Harmondsworth: Penguin. [Original work published 1962]

Calvino, I (1981) *If on a Winter's Night a Traveller*. London: Secker & Warburg.

Cooper, J (1986) *Riders*. London: Corgi.

Duguid, L (2002) Before it becomes literature. In Z Leader (ed), *On Modern British Fiction* (pp. 284–303). Oxford: Oxford University Press.

Eagleton, T (2005) *The English Novel: An introduction*. Oxford: Blackwell Publishing.

Golding, W (1957) *Lord of the Flies*. London: Faber. [Original work published 1954]

Greenberg, M (1971) *The Terror of Art: Kafka and modern literature*. London: Andre Deutsch.

Harris, R (1992) *Fatherland*. London: Hutchinson.

Harris, R (2006) *Imperium*. London: Hutchinson.

Hornstein, GA (2002) Narrative of madness as told from within. *The Chronicle Review*, 25 January, 7–10.

James, H (1963) *Portrait of a Lady*. Harmondsworth: Penguin. [Original work published 1875]

Johnson, BS (1969) *The Unfortunates*. London: Panther.

Joyce, J (1992) *Ulysses*. London: Penguin. [Original work published 1922]

Kafka, F (1933) *Metamorphosis*. London: Martin Secker & Warburg. [Original work published 1915]

Layard, R (2006) *The Depression Report*. London: London School of Economics.

Mantle, J (1989) *In for a Penny*. London: Sphere Books.

McEwan, I (2005) *Saturday*. London: Jonathan Cape.

Melville, H (2007) *Moby Dick*. Harmondsworth: Penguin Classics. [Original work published 1851]

Midgley, M (2001) *Science and Poetry*. London: Routledge.

Nabokov, V (1982) *Lectures on Literature*. London: Harvest.

Thirwell, A (2005) *Metamorphosis*. London: Vintage.

Tolstoy, L (1954) *Anna Karenina*. Harmondsworth: Penguin. [Originally published in serial form 1873–7]

Tolstoy, L (1957) *War and Peace*. Harmondsworth: Penguin Classics. [Originally published in serial form 1865–9]

Waugh, P (2005) Postmodern fiction and the rise of critical theory. In BW Shaffer (ed), *A Companion to the British and Irish Novel 1945–2000* (pp. 65–82). Oxford: Blackwell.

FICTION AND MADNESS

Tis strange – but true; for truth is always strange;
Stranger than fiction.
(Lord Byron, *Don Juan*)

Real world

At first sight writing a novel might seem a private even reclusive act. In fact, it's an endeavour that lends itself to considerations of sociality, economics and politics. Indeed, novelists seek to enlarge on these either in relation to themselves and/or, more expansively, to their immediate surroundings or nation-state. For instance, in *A Question of Power* (1974: 11; this volume, Chapter 12) Bessie Head describes one of her characters thus:

> It seemed almost incidental that he was African. So vast had his inner perceptions grown over the years that he preferred an identification with a particular environment. And yet, as an African, he seemed to have made one of the most perfect statements: 'I am just anyone'.

Such renderings of identity are rarely heard in the West today where 'self' has ceased to be about individual moral agency and more a self-aggrandising usage of 'rights' seemingly exercised with little attention to the effects on others. Working through this book, you will observe this 'self' ebb and flow in response to the twists and turns of politics, ethnicity, poverty, gender and affluence, that is, self as a product of its social time. You will also observe one of the few remaining situations where selfhood is routinely denied, namely when people are diagnosed mentally ill by a medical profession that claims independence from socio-political-cultural contingencies.

This is where fiction can help, by commenting on experiences that impinge on psychiatric practice and its effects on people's identities. Of course, the relative merits of the scientific versus the humanities is an argument going back to Plato who claimed that the productions of writers/artistes are no more than entertainments that actually mislead on questions about sanity. It is, he believed, to the scientific that we must turn for enlightenment about man's psychological status. This is a fair point but which has led, in our time, to reductive concepts of insanity and its treatment, and whilst it's true that 'the madman' in literature can be a 'literary device' intended to entertain, literary accounts highlight questions about insanity informatively but, as well, in ways that resonate with people because they are felt and understood intuitively.

In such ways, fiction complements scientific accounts, accentuating aspects that they fail to cover or don't cover at all. Robin Downie (2005: 49) contrasts concepts of 'pattern' and 'sequence' showing how scientific patterns, such as the double helix of DNA structure, are both temporal as well as inhabiting structured space, whereas sequences – events and human interactions – follow each other in time and, often uniquely so, in the lives of persons. We will confront this in the life of Bessie Head and her protagonist, Elizabeth, in *A Question of Power*. We will also see (Chapter 13) how sociologist Harold Garfinkel's (1967) research led to the discovery that people construct social worlds in sequences of time and space, thus expanding our understanding of personality. In effect, Garfinkel argues, people author themselves through living.

When reading a novel that addresses madness therefore, it will help to have 'some understanding, however shallow, of the period and context in which it was written, or else what it is talking about can easily escape us' (Moseley, 1989: 2). For instance, Mary McCarthy wrote *The Company She Keeps* (1942) contemporaneously with the rise of psychoanalysis. The psychoanalytic influence produced novels that broke from authorial interest in psychological character to ones where the characters *themselves* internalise and reflect on their motives, desires and beliefs. Phenomena such as psychological denial, repression, paranoia or the oedipal complex were hardly absent in literature up till then. However, now they appear less as clear story lines and more as conflicts to be worked through in the minds of the characters.

This emphasis subsequently changed when novelists began to perceive psychiatry as insufficient to explain or even describe behaviour. Eventually, novels such as Kingsley Amis's (1979) *Jake's Thing* (this volume, Chapter 4) or *One Flew Over The Cuckoo's Nest* (Kesey, 1973) would savage psychotherapies either as theoretically frivolous or as purveyors of intellectual oppression. Of course, by the time Amis wrote *Jake's Thing* psychoanalysis was on the wane anyway with behaviourism on the rise. Unsurprisingly therefore, Amis focuses mostly on the latter although he implies that *all* therapy is trite. In Kesey's novel, the character 'big nurse' conducts group therapy, the gold standard of the post-1970s Encounter movement, not as a means towards self-realisation but as a way of inducing psychological submission in a group of hospitalised male patients. This – the real point of the novel – is continually missed, most people opting for the lobotomy at the end of the story as the main iniquity.

Avoiding shallowness

In general, comparisons between the functions of literature and psychiatry can be made a tad too easily. Whereas psychiatry deals in predetermined categories of human action, confounding variables omitted, fiction insinuates irony, doubt, provocation, opening up, the inevitability of despair. The novel, says Shaffer (2005: xvii): 'is a genre that is ever questioning, ever examining itself and subjecting its established forms to review: it is the genre with most contact with the present (with contemporary reality) in all its open-endedness'. This is not to deny its utility as a psychological prism but that more so does it open up normative aesthetic and cultural roles from perspectives which encompass all, including psychiatric, claims to objectivity or truth.

At which point I confess that in order to make fiction's relevance more telling I have added two Shakespearian plays to my novel selections. My reason is that these plays superbly illustrate facets of psychopathic character, unpredictability and the role of evil in human nature and destiny. *Richard III* (this volume, Chapter 5), for instance, has warranted psychological analyses for years, Richard's actions deduced as compensation for physical deformity, the displacement of self-hatred on to others. Invoking Bessie Head's (this volume, Chapter 12) 'universal African' illuminates Richard's deformity not only as individual perversion but as devilish violation of the social order. His is personified evil warping an otherwise Utopian society, explicating Shakespeare's fear and disdain for civil disruption. So too do the Macbeths smell of evil with their disruption of the social and spiritual order of things. Here, murder is a compulsion shared by two persons comprised of one psychology, an obsessive craving for power corrupting them both, spinning them helplessly towards guilt, madness and suicide. 'Canst thou not minister to a mind diseas'd?' asks Macbeth of his doctor. The answer, for every successive generation, is revealing and salutary.

Ethnicity and culture

Understanding the socio-cultural background of fiction is germane when a writer's ethnic milieu markedly differs from our own. The novel's origins are in fact geographically miscellaneous and, outside England, examples of the form spurted in Russia, France, China, Ireland, Spain and, most recently, Africa and Asia. In respect of Africa, and to avoid the whiff of Eurocentrism, I include Bessie Head's *A Question of Power* (this volume, Chapter 12). Whilst an outstanding work on its own merits it also represents the postcolonial novel's examination of Africa's residual political and racial bitterness, albeit in this instance within a domain of madness. Elements of this also mediate another of my choices, *Felicia's Journey* (Trevor, 1994; this volume, Chapter 8) which itemises psychopathy, deceit and ethnic hatred against a backcloth of Irish-English history.

I turn now to Patrick McGrath's account of novel writing because he expands on what I've said so far and because his work explicates many of the issues that govern fiction writing's link to madness.

McGrath's fiction

McGrath believes that psychosis and writing are mutually exclusive, the one characterised by disintegration, the other 'yielding to a clear design'. So in *Asylum* (McGrath, 1997; this volume, Chapter 11) does he try to capture the chaotic nature and effects of psychotic actions. Actually, says Irish novelist William Trevor (Del Rio Alvaro, 2006: 120); see (this volume, Chapter 8): 'You *have* [my italics] to start with a mess, which is a bit like the mess we all live in in the world, you know. You start with that mess and you really have got to create this for yourself in your fiction.' Or, as Beckett succinctly puts it: 'to find a form that accommodates the mess, that is the task of the artist now' (Bair, 1978: 523).

To do this, novelists take autobiography as their starting point – the novelist is his/her own best instrument – and McGrath is no exception. His father was medical superintendent at Broadmoor Mental Hospital where McGrath lived from 1956 until 1981. As such, he knows mental hospitals from the inside, from the perspectives of staff *and* patients. Later on, working in a psychiatric unit, he again mingled with psychotic people but with a newfound ambition to seek:

> Some understanding, if such a thing were possible, of what gave rise to that thinking. I wanted, if I could, to seize upon some idea that would allow me an imaginative gateway in to the tortuous mazes of schizoid thinking.
> (McGrath 2002: 141)

This is important. Today's mental health workers are in the main, psychiatrists excepted, the offspring of empathy, genuineness and non-judgementalism. Carl Rogers (1967) and Abraham Maslow (1999) having arrived in the 1970s quickly became another orthodoxy, championing 'being with' and privileging other's experiences as the determinant of recovery. Thus did Roger's person-centredness begrudge psychotherapy of ideas replacing them with emotional 'conditions' which, until the arrival of aggressive CBT, occupied central place.

McGrath, however, argues that *ideas* are necessary to understanding psychiatric practice and that this trumps assertions that the emotional conditions that constitute 'encounters' between carers and patients are all that are required. Desiring to explain madness, McGrath read and read until he found a quote from anti-psychiatrist R.D. Laing (1960) (see Discussion Paper 1, pp. 189–91) that the schizophrenic 'is dying of thirst in a world of wet', that for mentally ill people there is but an appalling sense of solitude and incapacity. From this, McGrath wrote *Spider* (1991) in which symptoms medically defined as pathological are depicted as purposeful, as Spider's saving grace. With this novel, McGrath wants us to see that much of what has seemed bizarre and irrational can be made to fit into a coherent psychological pattern, a flawed and tragic pattern, to be sure, but a pattern nevertheless.

McGrath's 1997 *Asylum* (this volume, Chapter 11) is more elaborate in that staff as well as patients are accorded proportionate space. Remember, McGrath claims that describing the mind of 'the psychotic' is infinitely more challenging than that of 'normal' persons. But, as we will see, anxiety in everyone is exacerbated when barriers between staff and patients fracture, when institutional etiquette is transgressed. *Asylum* orchestrates the disintegration of a psychiatric social order almost comically unprepared to handle any violation of its rules.

Fiction's bedfellows

Some novelists bizarrely claim that they write for themselves and, when not pandering to common tastes, this is probably true. But it's a rare literary work that doesn't concern itself with its readers in some shape or form. For example, listen to novelist William Trevor (Del Rio Alvaro, 2006: 121): 'The reader is terribly, terribly important because without the reader, as far as I'm concerned, there's nothing. It's a kind of relationship, sometimes almost a friendship'. McGrath thinks that novels help us understand not just the experience of mental illness but how it impinges on people and social conventions. This doesn't demean the aesthetics of fiction but it places it within the practical concerns of readers and everyday life. Sylvia Plath's *The Bell Jar* (1963) for instance taps into the general socio-cultural background of its era, particularly the emergence of anti-psychiatry and feminism in the late 1960s and 1970s. Plath's novel is sometimes viewed as a critique of the mental institutions of its time, its mirroring of anti-psychiatric literature, for example Rosenhan's (1973) *On Being Sane in Insane Places* and texts by R. D. Laing (1960) and Thomas Szasz (1973) strongly supporting this. Indeed, Maria Farland (2002) argues that mental hospital closures were as much provoked by writers like Plath as by the radical psychiatric activists themselves. There may be something in this although cause–effect models of explanation are improbable where fiction is concerned. Plath's *The Bell Jar* is multifaceted and whilst it critiqued hospitals and their electroshock treatments, it also fixed a jaundiced eye on radical psychiatry's attitudes towards mental illness *and women*.

It is, in retrospect, a sobering thought that at the (in)famous 'Dialectics of Liberation Conference' (Cooper, 1968) neither female therapists nor political activists were involved other than – in the case of females – making the tea. Equally, the patients of radical psychiatrists were mainly women, male doctors posturing as philosopher kings and rescuer-salvationists. Plath's fiction acts on this, her protagonist Esther's treatment for depression depicted as a coercion into conformity. As an American, Plath brought a fresh perspective to social class and mental illness in England. She depicted radical psychiatry as a middle-class affair, the typical Laingian patient exhibiting remarkable articulation, distrust of conformity and sufficient wealth to buy radical (i.e. private) treatment, her protagonist Esther Greenwood embracing a private psychiatry unobtainable by working people. Not that class keeps male chauvinism at bay. Esther's boyfriend Buddy is an 'all American boy', an embodiment of intelligence, athleticism and he loves his mom's apple pie. He is everything a conventional well-educated American girl might want. But, as Esther quickly realises, he is also thoughtless, unable to understand her desire to write poetry and thus exist outside the coerciveness that marriage (to a Buddy) would bring. Esther reminisces (Plath, 1963: 89) how Buddy had once told her that having children would alter her creative designs, that the artistic impulse would sublimate within maternal love and wifely duty. For Esther, this sounds like some kind of programming into domestic subservience. This passage, in her novel, reminds you of Goffman's seminal text *Asylums* (1968) with its acerbic take on how behaviour is constructed through role pressures, some of which operate within time-honoured expectations. Plath knew of Goffman's critique and took a lead from it, forging an interdependency between literature and professional sociology. But mainly, *The Bell Jar* exemplifies how literature subjects psychiatry's ideas to broader intellectual control and the sobering effects of cultural artifice.

Some end points

If *The Bell Jar* is to be believed, little had changed in psychiatry, certainly for women, since the late nineteenth century when Charlotte Perkins Gilman (1899/ 1981) penned *The Yellow Wallpaper* (this volume, Chapter 6). With its account of women's subjection and neuroses (also expressed as a desire to write) Gilman's book was the starting point of rejection of masculinity feigning as benevolence and cure. Gilman's psychiatrist, Weir Mitchell, believes that sending women to bed for months without reading matter (thus preventing 'morbid thoughts' or wish fulfilment) is the way for them to go. So too in *The Bell Jar* is Esther, resisting conformist indices of womanhood, called 'neurotic' and 'crazy'.

This is not to homogenise women writers, their vision or literary ambitions. Pat Barker's *Regeneration* (1992, this volume, Chapter 3) for instance is largely populated by males and the hugely successful Margaret Atwood has influenced views about 'science fiction' defining her award-winning *The Handmaid's Tale* (1986) as 'speculative fiction, not to be confused with 'squids in the sky'. Duguid (2002: 296) also points out that some women writers, for example Barker, Rose Tremain, Jeanette Winterson and Hilary Mantel, had turned to historical fiction (in the 1980s) possibly to escape the intellectual tag, 'feminist novelists'.

Fiction's madness gifts us with insights that technical literature conceals or ignores. Apart from some dried-out ethical debates, psychiatric texts avoid crossovers from the personal to the professional and vice versa. Theirs is a parched, supposedly objective, emptied-out stance dogged in its conviction that meaning will ultimately coalesce under a microscope. With fiction, alternatively, there resides a capability, a power to engage with this supposition with every expectation that something more humanly recognisable will surface.

Professor John Shotter (1975), disturbed by psychology experiments that excluded experience, muttered of 'man buried beneath the debris of a million investigations'. It seems apposite to counter this, not from any wish to belittle 'the sciences' but to factor into distress its experiential base with, crucially, the subjection of this base to fictional exploration and control. My point is not to polarise theory and practice further but to explore how dissimilar thinking about madness materialised, how attitudes towards human, especially women's, mental status came about but mostly, to show how fiction's madness helps us better understand these things.

References

Amis, K (1979) *Jake's Thing*. Harmondsworth: Penguin.

Atwood, M (1986) *The Handmaid's Tale*. London: Cape.

Bair, D (1978) *Samuel Beckett: A biography*. London: Jonathan Cape.

Barker, P (1992) *Regeneration*. Harmondsworth: Penguin.

Byron, GG (1973) *Don Juan*. Harmondsworth: Penguin English Poets. [Original work begun in 1818]

Cooper, D (1968) *The Dialectics of Liberation*. Harmondsworth: Penguin.

Del Rio Alvaro, C (2006) Talking with William Trevor: It all comes naturally now. *Estudios Irlandeses, 1,* 119–24.

Downie, R (2005) Madness in literature: Device and understanding. In C Saunders & J Maclaughlin (eds) *Madness and Creativity in Literature and Culture* (pp. 49–63). Basingstoke: Palgrave Macmillan.

Duguid, L (2002) Before it becomes literature. In Z Leader (ed) *On Modern British Fiction* (pp. 284–303). Oxford: Oxford University Press.

Farland, M (2002) Sylvia Plath's anti-psychiatry. *Minnesota Review, 55,* 245–56.

Garfinkel, H (1967) *Studies in Ethnomethodology*. Cambridge: Polity Press.

Gilman, CP (1981) *The Yellow Wallpaper*. London: Virago. [Original work published 1899]

Goffman, E (1968) *Asylums: Essays on the social situation of mental patients and other inmates*. Harmondsworth: Penguin.

Head, B (1974) *A Question of Power*. London: Heinemann.

Kesey, K (1973) *One Flew Over the Cuckoo's Nest*. London: Picador. [Original work published 1962]

Laing, RD (1960) *The Divided Self*. London: Tavistock.

Maslow, AH (1999) *Toward a Psychology of Being*. Chichester: Wiley. [Original work published 1963]

McCarthy, M (1942) *The Company She Keeps*. Harmondsworth: Penguin.

McGrath, P (1991) *Spider*. New York: Vintage.

McGrath, P (1997) *Asylum*. London: Penguin.

McGrath, P (2002) Problem of drawing from psychiatry for a fiction writer. *Psychiatric Bulletin, 20,* 140–3.

Moseley, CWRD (1989) *Richard III*. Harmondsworth: Penguin.

Plath, S (1963) *The Bell Jar*. London: Faber.

Rogers, C (1967) *On Becoming a Person*. London: Constable.

Rosenhan, D (1973) On being sane in insane places. *Science, 179,* 250–8.

Shaffer, BW (2005) *The British and Irish Novel 1945–2000*. Oxford: Blackwell.

Shotter, J (1975) *Images of Man in Psychological Research*. London: Methuen.

Szasz, T (1973) *The Manufacture of Madness*. St. Albans: Paladin.

Trevor, W (1994) *Felicia's Journey*. London: Penguin.

CHAPTER 3

REGENERATION

What passing-bells for these who die as cattle?
Only the monstrous anger of the guns.
(Wilfred Owen, *Anthem for Doomed Youth*)

Pat Barker's *Regeneration* (1992) is set during the 1914–18 War, also known as
the First World War, also known as the Great War, where, it is worth remembering,
a soldier refusing to fight, or deemed to have left his post, would be court-
martialled and shot. Over 300 suffered this fate, nearly always following a cursory
trial, the executions carried out the next day at dawn. Unwillingness to fight (by
non-officers) therefore, was seen as treachery albeit treachery, that might entail
little more than stumbling back from the fight, distraught, traumatised, or having
lost one's rifle or sense of direction. As it was considered unthinkable that officers
be adjudged cowards, only a couple of these were shot and not before being
'broken down' in the ranks to non-officer status. Most officers were sent home
having been conceded some form of 'nervous debility' consequent on 'shell
shock' and so in need of treatment and recuperation: one such officer was the
poet Siegfried Sassoon.

Ⅰ   *Regeneration* covers the months July to November 1917 and is comprised of
historical as well as fictional characters. Amongst the former are W.H.R. Rivers,
an army psychiatrist, and Sassoon, a second lieutenant, one of a number of 1914–
18 soldiers known as 'the war poets'. Others of this group were Wilfred Owen,
Isaac Rosenberg, Edmund Blunden, Charles Hamilton Sorley and, perhaps most
famous of all, Rupert Brooke. Other conflicts, before and after, also produced
their poets but it is to the 1914–18 conflict that we turn for *the* pitiful, *the* pitiless
accounts of murderous guns, outright slaughter, wasted youth and on a scale never
seen before. The action of the novel takes place mainly at Craiglockhart Hospital,
a converted unit for the treatment of shell shock also known (within medical circles)
as neurasthenia (see Chapter 6 and Discussion Paper Five, pp. 202–4) and which
we would today call 'post-traumatic stress disorder'.

The effects of war

In general, the received wisdom is that events surrounding the Second World
War (1939–45) had a major effect on the practice of psychiatry in Britain. The
consensus has been that, prior to this, mental illness was seen by laymen, as

well as professionals, as inborn and irredeemable and thus reducible to biological and genetic explanation. It was a fault-line approach that excluded social and economic events. The psychological breakdowns of soldiers, who had entered the conflagration (of the Second World War) apparently sane, only to return 'broken men' led psychiatrists like Maxwell Jones (1982) to make connections between (war) trauma and its negative consequences. Jones' use of Da Costa's Syndrome advanced social psychology through the evolution of the 'therapeutic community' movement (Clarke, 2004) most famously at the Henderson Hospital. But in fact the roots of these changes go back further back than this and although, arbitrarily, one could go back as far as time allows, realistically the emergence of a humanitarian or social psychiatry, as against a strictly medical approach, came about from the events described in *Regeneration*.

Sassoon

Although decorated for heroism in the field, Siegfried Sassoon published a protest against the First World War (it is included at the beginning of the novel) in which he asserted that the politicians and military strategists of his own side were as responsible for the carnage as the enemy. This protest hit the headlines, was read out in Parliament, and could have resulted in his court-martial had not Sassoon's friend and fellow war poet, Robert Graves, author of *I Claudius*, intervened. Instead of a military court, disgrace and imprisonment, Sassoon was (dubiously) declared shell shocked and sent to Craiglockhart Hospital where he was treated by Dr. W.H.R. Rivers whose approach in no small way was influenced by Sigmund Freud (1995). It quickly transpires that Rivers doesn't see Sassoon as clinically ill, but does recognise, illness or no illness, that his war protest is problematic. This is because Rivers sees it as his duty – he is both psychiatrist and senior officer – to convince Sassoon that his protest is misplaced and that he must return to battle. Observe the interchanges (Barker, 1992: 73) when Rivers announces that his therapeutic sessions with Sassoon will be less frequent although still three times a week. When asked if that isn't a lot for someone who is 'not ill', Rivers replies: 'I shan't be able to persuade him to go back in less than that'. And he later adds: 'He's a mentally and physically healthy man. It's *his* duty to go back, and it's *my* [original italics] duty to see that he does.'

This raises a perennial conundrum of applied psychiatry, namely its socio-political as opposed to medical obligations and responsibilities and the manner by which it weights individual need against these broader requirements. It's as relevant a question today as it was then, the way in which some socially disruptive people are diagnosed as mentally ill, subsequently detained and treated.

Class and gender

Not only a student of Freudian psychology, Rivers was also schooled in anthropology. That being so, he approached mental trauma as both unconscious phenomenon and as an outcome of relentless stress, in this instance the terrors of warfare. In the case of neurasthenia, Rivers knew that current medical thinking recognised social stress as a precursor but that this was typically a (peacetime) explanation applied to females. Rivers, however, had begun to conceive of the social dimension as a way of explaining the pathological reactions of soldiers exposed to sustained artillery fire, a considerable extension of the theory in gendered terms.

Not that this shift in thinking applied to 'the men', those lower in the ranks. Rather was it reserved for those of higher military status (and class). Freud himself had doubted if psychoanalysis could be of use to 'the working man' restricting it to those sufficiently educated and capable of intellectual reflection. Rivers had noted that mutism, a common reaction to stress:

> seemed to spring from a conflict between *wanting* [original italics] to say something, and knowing that if you *do* [original italics] say it the consequences will be disastrous. So you resolve it by making it physically impossible for yourself to speak. And for the private soldier the consequences of speaking his mind are always going to be far worse than they would be for an officer. What you tend to get in officers is stammering ... all the physical symptoms: paralysis, blindness, deafness, are all common in private soldiers and rare in officers. It's almost as if for the labouring classes illness *has* [original italics] to be physical.
> (Barker, 1992: 96)

To what extent was this true? Which is to say, *actually* true as opposed to a product of class-obsessed perception? Could it still be true? You might wish to consider if class still identifies people who enter psychotherapy, bearing in mind that the latter is now largely a privately financed enterprise. Does the language of therapy/counselling presuppose particular levels/types of education in its clients? Are levels of emotional need/beliefs similar between clients and counsellors? Do they share some form of dedication to psychologising everyday life?

Freud

Remember that Freudian theory took shape from concepts (and treatments) of female hysteria (formulated by male doctors). Rivers' distaste for physical treatments and his willingness to understand patients' problems marked him out (professionally) as controversial and, in the eyes of some, a 'soft touch' for manipulative, self-serving patients. Observe Rivers' *attitudes* towards Sassoon (Barker, 1992: 115):

> As soon as you accepted that the man's breakdown was a consequence of his war experience rather than of his innate weakness, then inevitably the war became the issue, and the therapy was a test, not only of the genuineness of the individual's symptoms but also of the validity of the demands that war was making of him.

This surpasses medical psychiatry by embracing 'the social' as salient, that the social carries explanatory weight not just within normative, peacetime conditions but in war as well. That social indices underscored mental distress was later reinforced by Brown and Harris (1978) whose work contested medical descriptions of depression. Itemising specific needs in young mothers, they demonstrated that economic deprivation could induce severe depression. Smail (1993) has (more persistently) outlined the negative effects of environments on mental health insisting that any understanding of psychological distress that didn't assess how market forces disenfranchise poor and/or deprived people was insufficient. The question then turns on *who* is secure, *who* is disadvantaged, *who* is alienated and, how does deprivation unbalance mental health.

Although Rivers published papers on Freudian psychology he was sceptical of the sexual symbolism in Freud's work, a scepticism which stemmed from his training in anthropology. It was anthropology in fact that nudged him towards an ecological view of mental breakdown. In this, he becomes the perfect device for examining war neuroses both as psychological *and* social phenomena. The point is, psychiatry is not an objective entity and war highlights this. For example, questions of duty prevail, of obligation (towards self and others), of honour, country, history. Dr Yealland's approach denies this, reducing matters to physicality which he seeks to treat with electricity and burning. Barker might have made Yealland her protagonist and it's a toss-up as to the kind of difference that would have made to *Regeneration*. Yet it is Rivers and Sassoon, together, who became the point of comparison and departure for the novel's other characters and events. The fact is, Rivers' philosophical position enables Barker to pepper the novel with psychoanalytic motifs of various sorts. Chapter four, for instance, begins with Anderson, one of Rivers' patients, relating a dream that is jam-packed with Freudian symbols albeit a difficulty arises when Anderson, a medical doctor, resists River's psychoanalytic interpretations. For Anderson, Rivers' questions about the meaning of 'the post mortem apron' are redolent of: 'what you Freudian Johnnies are on about all the time' (Barker, 1992: 29).

From its beginnings, psychoanalysis was resented by organic, conventional psychiatrists because it challenged positivism and biological legitimacy. Yet much as they might wish, they could hardly claim immunity from the psychoanalytic claim that behaviour is unconsciously determined. It's an (ongoing) tension, well captured by Yealland and Rivers, the distinction sustained today between a reinvigorated positivism which sits uncomfortably alongside the prizing, by some, of the (sometimes accusatory) narratives of clients concerning their treatment and its outcomes.

A male malady

Rivers' recognised an ongoing reciprocity between war and distress (Barker, 1992: 222). He knew that it was: 'prolonged strain, immobility and helplessness that did the damage, and not the sudden shocks or bizarre horrors that the patients themselves were inclined to point to as the explanation for their condition'. This link however had previously been seen as a psychological dependency inbred in the physical *and* psychological make-up of women. *Regeneration* uses this idea to reassess the potential vulnerability of men under conditions of war that had vastly reduced their autonomy, indeed *any* sense of their being in control.

Enticed by the 'glory' of war, anticipating a 'boy's own' escapade that will qualify them as men, the youth of 1914 find themselves stuck in stinking trenches, up to their knees in mud next to their comrade's skulls, awaiting death's turn (see Barker's description of trench life, 1992: 102–4). For many at the time, beliefs about war were impossibly romantic, an adventure in search of an ideal, tears vying with pride as they wrote and read their war poems. Read Rupert Brooke's resigned, tragic, lines (1918: 'The Soldier'): 'If I should die, think only this of me: / That there's some corner of a foreign field / That is forever England ...' lines whose innocence quickly congealed to horror and disbelief. But at first there was only imminent glory as Tommy Atkins went to fight with great expectations, knowing he would soon be back home. A popular song, written in 1914 by Ivor Novello and Lena Ford, was:

Keep the home fires burning
While your hearts are yearning,
Though your lads be far away they dream of home.
There's a silver lining, through the dark clouds shining
Turn the dark cloud inside out, 'till the boys come home'.

The tone is sentimental but optimistic, the prospect of war daunting but ultimately capable of being overcome. When Lord Kitchener initially called for 100,000 volunteers, within a single week ending September 1914 he got 175,000 and by the end of the month three quarters of a million. Little did they know that he was calling them to a plague.

At Craiglockhart

Although war may imminently kill them, yet do Sassoon and the others tread their way through a narrative dotted with social and political upheaval, a class-based psychiatry and homoeroticism.

Rivers believes that he can help patients by bringing a sense of himself into their therapy, perhaps as a kind of father figure. The image of fatherhood is important in the novel (Barker, 1992: 34-35, 65) principally because many who were about to die were conscious of not being fathers, of never having had, even, an intimate sexual encounter. Rivers wants to be their mentor and although often provoked by them, he remains outwardly empathetic. As you read his conversations with Sassoon, what do they say, in a professional sense, about him? From your knowledge of Freud's psychology, does Rivers pursue a strictly Freudian line with Sassoon or with any of his other patients?

A sexuality of passivity is palpable here: the men's self-esteem has been shot to pieces and Rivers suspects that vulnerability, previously identified as exclusively female, lies behind this. A good (if flawed) book to read at this point is Elaine Showalter's *Hystories* (1998), especially chapter two, which shows how hysteria was either camouflaged in 'real men' or otherwise linked to effeminacy or homosexuality. Homosexual references (Barker, 1992: 70, 98) occur throughout *Regeneration*, for instance where Rivers intently watches two male patients scything grass, stripped to the waist. Reprimanded by a senior officer, the two men begin to re-dress: 'Slowly, they reached for their uniforms, pulled khaki shirts and tunics on to sweating bodies, buckled belts. It had to be done though it seemed to Rivers that the scything went more slowly after that, and there was less laughter which seemed a pity.'

Look also at Barker's description of officers and men: 'mobilized into holes in the ground so constricted they could hardly move' (Barker, 1992: 107), a homoeroticism of brutal, close, physical contact. Also, what does Rivers mean when he says that he 'wished he was young enough for France'? And again, (Barker, 1992: 116) captivated by a young waiter, he tells how: 'It was possible to see the nape of his neck, defenceless under the stiff collar.' On the next page, we discover Sassoon also looking at the boy, the sort of boy, they agree, who would make a nice servant, to which Rivers adds: 'Not bad-looking either.'

But it runs deeper than this. Rivers knows that asking young patients to abandon repression, to come to terms with emotions conventionally despised in males, is asking a lot. But he has to pressure them if they are to face vulnerability, not as a prelude to the efficacy of his treatment, but as a baseline from which to usher them back to the fight.

Regeneration examines the conflicts that war and duty engender and how these impact on mental well-being, not only in relation to 'patients' but for all of those involved. For example, as his talks with Sassoon proceed, Rivers begins to examine his own position about the war, slowly acknowledging its terrible effects, its destructiveness in *every* respect and the powerlessness of psychology to account for such a catastrophe.

Psychiatry, fiction, history

Fiction constructs itself around character and so, here, we feel the horribleness of war more than a thousand historical/academic accounts could ever convey. Narrative also informs us how to work out meaningful responses to people mentally damaged by armed and/or violent conflict. The principles that lay behind Sassoon's treatment heralded the development of therapeutic communities with their psychosocial orientation to mental distress, its origins and treatment. That said, it would take a Second World War (a mere 21 years later) to solidify evidence that psychological disorder was not necessarily hereditary. Pioneers like Maxwell Jones (who founded the Henderson Therapeutic Community in 1947) quickly realised that beliefs about mental illness as biologically inherent could hardly explain the positive correlations between psychological distress and battle.

This was yet to come however, matters being dealt with very differently in the 1914–18 War with attitudes resolutely tied to ideals of chivalry, manliness, class and where violating these was seen as cowardice or madness. So was Sassoon confined to a hospital, his protest seen as a consequence of mental illness, a harsh enough judgement but whose fate would have been much worse had he been a working-class man or been assigned to Yealland as his doctor.

The poems

At this point, read Sassoon's (1947) war poetry and try to get a feel for his protest, his disillusionment. Equally, read Wilfred Owen (1963), also hospitalised at Craiglockhart and, in this instance, dreadfully shell shocked. The greatest of the war poets, Owen enters the novel about a quarter way through, a stammering, dark-haired boy asking Sassoon for his autograph. He is enamoured of Sassoon's good looks, the clipped aristocratic voice, bored expression, natural arrogance and the reputation for courage. Yet when they discuss poetry, Owen's stammer recedes and they talk of war as timeless, *ancient*, as if the present conflict is ahistorical so that survival is all that may be achieved: that is, war will happen again, and again.

Sassoon's later war poems differed greatly from Brooke's elegiac 'think only this of me' written at the War's start. Not that the change was entirely chronological. When Charles Hamilton Sorley fell at Loos in 1915 these lines were found on his person:

When you see millions of the mouthless dead
Across your dreams in pale battalions go,
Say not soft things as other men have said
That you'll remember. For you need not so.

This sonnet, says Martin Stephen (1993: 28), 'may have been written as a direct rebuttal of Brooke's patriotic sonnets. Sorley was certainly familiar with Brooke's work, and found himself very much at odds with the sentiments Brook expressed in the patriotic sonnets.'

Like Sorley, only later, Sassoon's beliefs about war became calloused. Whereas initially he had flung himself into battle, the hideousness of trench death strengthened his resolve to convey this to the British public. In this, he was influenced by Owen's belief in the senselessness of this absurdly ineffectual (geographical) war of attrition. (In one battle alone, the Somme, there were 420,000 British casualities, almost 20,000 killed on the first day of an offensive that lasted from July till November 1916. As a result of this battle, British forces gained approximately 12 kilometres of pot-holed ground called 'no-man's land'.) It was this that led Owen to produce his most scathing poems and it is these that we remember and celebrate so well. Yet the bravery of these young volunteers, and their sacrifice, is also captured in the letters of those less educated, the so-called 'men', the other 95 per cent. Here, Private George Morgan (1976), who fought at the Somme, remembers:

> There was no lingering about when zero hour came. Our platoon officer blew his whistle and he was the first up the scaling ladder, with his revolver in one hand and a cigarette in the other. 'Come on boys,' he said, and up he went. We went up after him one at a time. I never saw the officer again. His name is on the memorial to the missing which they built after the war at Thiepval. He was only young but he was a very brave man.

Even here, the whiff of class superiority presides, the private as follower, the young officer, cigarette in hand, charging at the front. Although just as brave, the 'working man', it seems, didn't do 'dashing'.

Why did Sassoon protest?

What do you learn about Sassoon's disdain for war as you read his poems? Are his attitudes towards war a product of mental illness and, allowing that this was believed by many at the time, what does that reveal about attitudes towards mental illness in 1917? Opinion was divided within the military, a minority conceding a concept of shell shock – initially ascribed to a *physical* alteration in the ear or brain brought on by gas or the roar of the guns – but with most preferring to see shocked reactions as cowardice and deserving a firing squad.

An additional light is thrown on this in that government ministers lied about the executions to Parliament. It might be they feared a general outcry if the executions become widely known. General Haigh, who signed the death warrants, lied when he said that each man had been medically examined prior to execution. Indeed, only recently has a truer picture emerged, that most of those shot *were* shell shocked and in no position (and with little assistance) to contest desertion charges or to appeal their death sentences. In effect, the executions, as was their purpose, served as a warning, a deterrent to others not to run shy of the guns. In Joseph Losey's (1964) film *King and Country,* Private Hamp receives a 'Dear John' letter from his missus. Three years in the trenches, he has lost all his mates to the blasted guns. Following a huge bombardment he decides enough is enough and sets out to 'walk home to England'. Detained at Calais, an army doctor refuses to diagnose 'shell shock' and he is shot 'pour encourarger les autres' (to encourage the others). It is a haunting film of misery wrapped in cruelty and human disregard. It's also an exercise in who gets what as a function of class and social position. Hamp is a working-class man who volunteered, perhaps blindly, for 'King and Country'. Those around him, those who condemn as well as those who try to help him, know a great deal more about (the) war and its cynical origins, even if they can't prevent his death. Rules are rules: he had his duty to do and he didn't do it.

Forms of address

On the question of social class, observe how Pryor, Sassoon and Rivers address each other. Pryor, a fictional character, is unwilling to see Rivers as a father figure and, in their discussions, he delights in obfuscation, cynicism and verbal aggression. Part of Rivers' difficulty is that he recognises, in Pryor's behaviour, his own problems with authority figures. But note as well how class intervenes. Pryor, as perceived by Rivers, is not *quite* officer material and he knows that Rivers thinks this. Rivers calls him *Mister* Pryor whereas Sassoon quickly becomes Siegfried and who, in turn, calls Rivers by his surname, a felicity often employed by the upper classes. And when Pryor questions Rivers about mutism in officers, Rivers replies:

> Mutism seems to spring from a conflict between *wanting* to say something and knowing that if you *do* say it the consequences will be disastrous. So you resolve it by making it physically impossible for yourself to speak. And for the private soldier the consequences of speaking his mind are always going to be far worse than they would be for an officer. What you tend to get in officers is stammering. And it's not just mutism. All the physical symptoms: paralysis, blindness, deafness. They're all common in private soldiers ... Its almost as if for the ... labouring classes illness *has* to be physical.
> (Barker, 1992: 96, all italics original)

And class also permeates many encounters that take place beyond the predominantly military/medical setting of the novel. Watch Pryor distance himself from Sarah when he suspects her of reading too much into their relationship, how he tells her a story (Barker, 1992: 131) about censorship and class in the army. Pryor's sexual status is ambiguous here and we realise early on that he is not fully heterosexual. And so a mosaic of themes, events and characters emerge in ways that seem contemporary (to us) even though set in a particular time and place. We are reminded again of the class-based origins of psychotherapy and its ongoing utility to educated, affluent and self-inquisitive people.

Summary

Rivers is a psychiatrist but he is also part of a war machine. Therefore his loyalty to his patients is twofold; he is their doctor *and* their senior officer. This complicates his treatment since his duty is to convince them that their war protest is mistaken. The tension of this is played out in his efforts to 'cure' Siegfried Sassoon, an officer and a gentleman who is virulently anti-war but who is, as well, (supposedly) suffering from shell shock. Believing that Sassoon is not ill makes it easier for Rivers to convince him of the error of his ways. The novel ends with Sassoon returning to active duty. In fact, he survived the war dying a week before his 81st birthday in 1967. Most of the other war poets fared less well. Charles Hamilton Sorley was killed by a sniper at the Battle of Loos, aged 20. Wilfred Owen was killed at the Battle of Sambre: he was 25. His mother received news of his death as her local church bells chimed the War's end. Edmund Blunden survived, dying in 1974 aged 78. He had become professor of poetry at Oxford University. Isaac Rosenberg was killed either in close combat or by a sniper at the Somme: he was 28. Rupert Brooke, en route to Gallipoli, died from septicaemia caught from a mosquito bite: he too was 28.

That *Regeneration* includes non-fictional characters that were there helps evoke the terribleness of the war. But *Regeneration* is not history. Rather does it re-*create* a cataclysmic 'event' which:

> asks readers to consider remembering as a form of healing, as a way to regenerate the bodies and the minds damaged by body politic. By locating the war's sins in the laws of society rather than the laws of nature, Barker offers a method of healing available not just to The Lost Generation, but to contemporary ones.
> (Westman, 2001: 60)

But precisely who or what is regenerated? Is it Sassoon and the others who return to battle? Or is *Regeneration* about condemning war as reprehensible and demeaning? Is it the blood sacrifice of the young that drapes nations in ever greater glory? Important too is the question of *how* regeneration comes about, the means by which ends are achieved. For Rivers, the problem was how best to understand psychological distress and apply right ways of treating it. Towards the novel's end we confront Dr Yealland's aggressive, if more 'scientific', treatments. Averse to psychologising, Yealland regards shellshock as a deviance from duty, a cowardice. Immune to the ethics of 'means justifying ends' Yealland uses electroshock to successfully rid an officer of mutism. Witnessing this, Rivers realises that both he and Yealland silence patients in the name of a higher force. Their methods differ but their aims are the same. And to top it all, Rivers is about to send a man to probable death in a war that he, Rivers, is now less sure about, musing that: 'A society that devours its own young deserves no automatic or unquestioning allegiance' (Barker, 1992: 249). Cocooning the action in and around Craiglockhart Hospital strengthens the war's effects because it centres and intensifies the characters' experiences and memories. Whereas Sebastian Faulkes' *Birdsong* (1994) takes a panoramic view of trench warfare, perceiving the horrors as inherent in human nature, Barker's vision is grounded in sociality, tied into man-made explanations, incomplete perhaps, but all the more tragic for that.

Currently, we espouse reductionist approaches to mental health problems. With much gusto, reinvented biological-genetic explanations of behaviour prevail, and with a pharmacological industry eagerly in tow. Further, we are admonished to attend to only that for which material evidence exists, to disallow what may be seen as rhetorical or speculative. But we have learned from *Regeneration* that ends, whatever their nature or quality, do *not* justify means. As we read our way through Yealland's treatment of the patient Callan, we realise that however 'successful' the 'therapy', a seam of humanity has been burned out of the soldier *and his therapist* in the process.

Without wishing to disown physical interventions entirely, construing the origins of mental illness devoid of sociality, ethics and human agency is risky. Today, a small window of hope, we accept psychiatric service users as co-participants. They are the heirs of 'the therapeutic community', the culmination of 'the community as doctor', something life enhancing that arose (strangely) from the conflagration of war.

Postscript

In no circumstances whatever will the expression 'shell-shock' be used verbally or be recorded in any regimental or other casualty report or in any hospital
or other medical document.
  (British Army General Routine Order No. 2384, issued on 7 June 1917)

Films

Regeneration was directed by Gillies MacKinnon for BBC Pictures. It received only a limited release and was not a hit. It opened to mixed reviews, some critics seeing it as over-romanticising war whilst others viewed the script as arch and overly grounded in technical discussion. It has, as you would expect from a British production, excellent performances with James Wilby as Sassoon and Jonathan Pryce as W.H.R. Rivers. Its depiction of the trenches is exceptional and we are not spared the horror and its effects on the mental health of the soldiers. The latter is one of the films special points in that most war films ignore how the terror lingers in the minds of its victims.

King and Country was a small-budget film directed by Joseph Losey in 1964. It addresses issues of war and duty and is, as well, emblematic of how class permeates military and judicial systems and, by implication, English society. The part of Private Hamp is played by Tom Courtenay whose performance deservedly won awards and Dirk Bogarde is the defending officer/lawyer. The drama brilliantly conveys how 'the individual' must be sacrificed to the (perceived) greater need of maintaining morale and winning a war, even as humanly degrading a war as this.

References

Barker, P (1992) *Regeneration*. Harmondsworth: Penguin.

Brooke, R (1918) *The Collected Poems*. London: Sidgwick.

Brown, GW & Harris, T (1978) *The Social Origins of Depression*. London: Tavistock.

Clarke, L (2004) *The Time of the Therapeutic Communities*. London: Jessica Kingsley Publishers.

Faulkes, S (1994) *Birdsong*. London: Vintage.

Freud, S (1995) *New Introductory Lectures on Psychoanalysis*. New York: W.W. Norton.

Jones, M (1982) *The Process of Change*. London: Routledge & Kegan Paul.

Losey, J (1964) *King and Country* [Film]. London: BHE Films.

MacKinnon, G (1997) *Regeneration* [Film]. UK: Artificial Eye.

Morgan, G (1976) *Private Morgan Interview*. Available online at: *http://uktv.co.uk/history/item/aid/571340*

Owen, W (1963) *The Collected Poems*. London: Chatto.

Sassoon, S (1947) *Collected Poems*. London: Faber.

Showalter, E (1998) *Hystories*. London: Picador.

Smail, D (1993) *The Origins of Unhappiness*. London: HarperCollins.

Stephen, M (1993) *Poems of the First World War*. London: Dent.

Westman, K (2001) *Regeneration: A reader's guide*. London: Continuum.

JAKE'S THING

If you can't annoy somebody with what you write, I think there is little point in writing.

So said Kingsley Amis whose first novel *Lucky Jim* (1961) established him as the finest comic novelist of the late twentieth century or even the finest novelist. Although he subscribed to the realist tradition in fiction *Jake's Thing,* his 1979 novel, may be taken generally as a social satire, a literary work to be sure, but with lots to say about its times and, especially, psychiatry in the 1970s. A complex and difficult man, Amis was plagued by phobias and fears. He had a horror of the dark and of being alone (except when writing) and had flown in an aeroplane, *once.* His contemporaries regarded him as an outstanding raconteur: 'above all quick-minded, verbally agile, terribly funny, a vigorous persecutor of bores, pseuds and wankers and a most tremendous mimic' (Jacobs, 1995b: 28).

He occasionally brought mimicry into his fiction. In *Lucky Jim*, the Jim in question uncontrollably and unconsciously pulls faces behind his colleague's backs and in *You Can't Do Both* (1994), one of Amis's friends appears as Jeremy Carpenter who turns:

> out to be a wonderful mimic. He makes the Dons sound like senile idiots, as in Amis's much admired impersonation of Lord David Cecil: 'I want you all to wemembah …'. He makes funny faces, including a killing upper-class moron face with a lot of blinking and as many as possible of the lower teeth showing.
> (Leader, 2006: 81)

As for Jacob's allusion to Amis's dislike of poseurs, the following appears in Amis's *Memoirs* (1992: 321). Taken to dinner by an American writer called Leo Rosten, they visit a 'trattoria-type restaurant' where:

> Rosten put on a revolting pseudo-Italian show of delighted cries and embraces with the proprietor and the waiter and doubtless others too … he was turning out to be nearly the sort of American who tells you that in the United States we have this man we call the president.

Memoirs is a series of pen-portraits of luminaries whom Amis had met across his lifetime. What's telling is that of the 26 characters he chose to write about only two were women, whom he admired, although the Mrs Thatcher chapter does contain a reservation or two. This says something about Amis's complex attitudes towards females. Although, in the memoirs, he lacerates his male subjects every one, his was nevertheless a man's world to which women could be admitted but on his terms. In addition to women, the kind of things that 'wound him up' seem whimsical for a man of otherwise fine judgement. Favourite irritations included people who (a) are tight-fisted and especially (b) don't buy their round, (c) are patronising, (d) self-effacing, falsely modest or pretentious and if any of these were inapplicable, there was always the catch-all category 'bore'.

A required word about women

Although a legendary womaniser, Amis was sardonic about women all told and more so as he grew older. The term misogynist – one who hates women – could have been invented for him. Yet he genuinely loved his first wife Hilly and rued the day he left her. Curiously, she would return to him (accompanied by an aristocrat, and penniless, husband) as his paid housekeeper. An oddish ménage à trois (and utterly non-sexual) it wasn't without its tensions, but it worked. In general Amis believed that whilst *some* women had talent, most didn't and, as we shall see, such are the attitudes of Jake Richardson, the protagonist of *Jake's Thing*. Indeed, with age, Amis's Blimpish outlook embraces a growing number of targets, typically passing fads and fancies, what we would nowadays call 'political correctness'. Something of his thinking is gleaned from an unfinished, untitled, poem in which he imbued women, 'queers' and children with emotional weaknesses unlike men who, though they may experience anguish, are still the ones to the forefront, managing life unbowed. Whilst such views are a (sore) point in themselves, what's interesting is the extent to which Amis may have tempered them when writing his novels.

That is, is *Jake's Thing* a conduit for the sneers, angst and bullishness of an ageing and disappointed (in love, in life) man? This question will work its way through this book, whether a writer's autobiography impinges on his/her fiction. And if, as I suspect it does, then should such intrusions remain hidden and if they don't, does the result still count as fiction? Fictional elements appear in all writing, the issue being one of control, the degree to which a writer constrains his biography *within* characterisation and story.

Jake's Thing

Jake's Thing was published when Amis's marriage (his second) to the novelist Elizabeth Jane Howard was falling apart after eighteen years (see Howard's (2002) account of this) and with Amis (so he said) wondering what he'd ever seen in her. In truth, she had grown weary of him, dismayed at the way he portrayed her in his novels as well as at his drinking which grew so bad as he grew older that more often than not he crawled to bed on all fours. He knew that to stop drinking, as she wanted him to, would have made him hate her all the more, and more quickly. But, drink or no drink, he wrote and wrote: no matter how dreadful the hangover he was at the typewriter every morning, churning out measured amounts, steadily watching his novels build and build.

By the late 1970s, his libido (he detested the 'Italian' pronunciation *libeeedo*) was deserting him and for someone of heretofore gluttonous sexual appetite, this probably bugged him. Classically, the psychiatric literature describes loss of libido as the downside of alcoholism. Shakespeare's take on this (in Macbeth) marks Amis's position well:

Macduff: What three things does drink especially provoke?
Porter: Marry sir, nose-painting, sleep and urine. Lechery sir, it provokes and unprovokes; it provokes the desire, but it takes away the performance; therefore, much drink may be said to be an equivocator with lechery: it makes him, and it mars him; it sets him on, and it takes him off; it persuades him, and disheartens him; makes him stand to, and not stand to; in conclusion, equivocates him in a sleep, and, giving him the lie, leaves him.
(Act II, sc iii, 26–30)

How to interpret this? The porter is drunk as he speaks and so must know what he's talking about! 'Equivocates him in a sleep' refers to dreams of a sexual nature but which simply lead to waking up and the need to pee. Don't be scared by the 'warts and all' imagery in the Shakespeare quote, it echoes the contradictory miseries of hard drinking, the horrors it brings, not just physically, nose picking depicting the bulbous red nose of the binger, but also psychologically, as in maritally and socially. Not for nothing do male alcoholics displace their self-loathing onto their partners, screaming infidelity when, in fact, these are the projections of self-disgust, impotence, isolation, apprehension and infidelity with the bottle.

But is psychologising sufficient in these cases or do we gain something more from fiction, from imagination, fantasy and creativity? Certainly it would be a mistake to see *Jake's Thing* in strictly autobiographical terms. Although, like other novelists, Amis conceded that his life was discernable in his work, this just acknowledges, unavoidably if you think about it, that all fiction stems from human experience, that in writing fiction, the 'facts' of experience are reconstructed through the imagination of love, malice and much else. In doing this, novelists must not show their hand *too* much and if, as happens, speeches or 'messages' sprout from the mouths of thinly drawn characters, then the novel, or the play, forfeits its best asset, which is to subject reality to creative revision. Here is Amis's son Martin, also a novelist, commenting on *Jake's Thing* which he sees as too close to his father's life:

I wasn't making the elementary error of conflating the man and the work, but all writers know that the truth *is* in the fiction. That's where the spiritual thermometer gives its reading. And Kingley's novels, around then, seemed to me in moral retreat, as if he were closing down a whole dimension – the one that contained women and love.

(Amis, 2000: 230)

The resemblance of Amis to Jake, said the son, was 'asphyxiatingly close' even if it faded in his later work. Martin Amis believed that it was his mother's return that rekindled humanity in his father, a humanity that subsequently led to novels that lanced hatred of self, of women, of life, the hatreds that so infected *Jake's Thing*. However, that, as we shall see, would come later. The following encapsulates Jake's views about women.

Their concern with the surface of things, with objects and appearances, with their surroundings and how they looked and sounded in them, with seeming to be better and to be right whilst getting everything wrong, their automatic assumption of the role of injured party in any clash of wills, their certainty that a view is the more credible and useful for the fact that they hold it, their use of misunderstanding and misrepresentation as weapons of debate, their selective sensitivity to tones of voice, their unawareness of the difference in themselves between sincerity and insincerity ... their fondness for general conversation and directionless discussion, their pre-emption of the major share of feeling ... their never listening.

And this comes at the novel's end (p. 286). There's a lot more venom leading up to it. The impression is of someone recognising interdependency between the sexes but who remain, still, incompatible. Most would find such views psychologically immature and/or socially limiting not only in strictly gendered terms but morally and politically as well. That they are compensated for by a fictional subtlety that lends them a 'possibility of truth' may be difficult to accept but is true nevertheless. It may be imperialistic but the world of fiction works outside everyday restrictions, it's a 'make believe' that asks you to believe in and take from it. Says Samuel Beckett (1986): 'Nothing matters but the writing. There has been nothing else worthwhile ... a stain upon the silence.'

Amis believed that women writers couldn't do this, that they were congenitally unable to go beyond expressing emotion, to concentrate on the problems and styles of communication itself. This didn't prevent his engaging with and even admiring some of the women whom he had come to know across his life. However he had come to 'know' a much greater number of women carnally such that even with those for whom he felt love, the sexual element was central.

Growing old

Amis wrote *Jake's Thing* in his fifties. As a young man his politics were to the Left (he had once been a communist of sorts!) but, with age, he drifted (as do most) to the Right. Ultimately he delighted in Margaret Thatcher – except on issues of higher education which, he believed, were belittled by university expansion with its consequent lowering of standards. It was Amis who coined the phrase 'more will mean less', that increasing college places would reduce the quality of education with a concomitant decrease in the calibre of graduates. To this day, proponents and opponents of university expansion call up his 'more will mean less' as the phrase that best captures the tension of the argument.

But, in general, his support of right-wing political agendas proceeded more as a protest against radicalism and fashionableness, his being the quiet, neurotic, conservatism that abhors change, suspecting it as usually being for its own sake. Also fearing the future, Amis keeps his self to himself, struggling against the demands of his surroundings at every possible level.

The novel

The early chapters unfold from Jake's perspective. That being the case, you might try building a profile of him bearing in mind the crumbling traditional values and social decay that are the (perceived) conditions against which he struggles. This is a man 'gone cold' on life, 'society' has left him high and dry, marginalised him by its abandonment of high culture and the values of intelligence and discernment. He has acquired a talent for diligence when in the company of others, generally taking the form of wanting to get by. You can hear Jake's attitudes in the talk of those people 'who don't want any trouble' or who just 'want to keep their heads down'. Jake's problem is that life won't let him be, so that he is occasionally impelled to hit back albeit, in his wife's case, with circumspection. In her presence, best to err on the side of quietude and not say *too* much, even when *knowing* that she is wrong. She, of course, is Everywoman: living, breathing, proof that females are aliens, necessary across a range of fronts of course but not like men, indeed *not* men. Which is not to say *inferior*, for they are to be feared both for their capacity to deny the obvious as well as that special ability to instil guilt via silence and, of course, that inherent, endless, predisposition to umbrage. Like Amis, Jake too has lost the urge for sex: no longer driven to possess women in this way, it may be that the drabness he sees everywhere reflects the one thing that fuelled all else, gave things their purpose.

What do you think?

Is Jake someone to admire, like, love, loathe, fear, ignore? Though we would today call him 'politically incorrect', does it follow that *all* of his fears and loathing are culpable? Are not some of his pet hates fair game, such as:

> his horror of imitation wrought-iron gates, or the way that saying 'please'
> can be made to sound rude, or busses that expect you to have the EXACT
> fare and shops which announce 'ten pence off EVERYTHING' but when
> paying for your chocolates are told, 'not ciggies or chocolates'.
>   (Amis, 1979: 14)

We could all add to these: radio advertisements, for instance, that flourish their wares only to end with fiercely accelerating voiceovers that 'the offer is subject to conditions' or that 'restrictions may apply'. To Amis's pique at verbal exchanges which end in 'cheers' we can add those sentences that end with an upwardly ascending vocal pitch. But, above all, there is Jake's suppressed vexation at the verbal dexterities of psychotherapists. Agonise with him, if you will, when he so wants to be sat in his favourite armchair watching *The Bill* but can't because he is caught up in the inane babblings of a group-work facilitator, Ed, and his acolytes as they postulate the untested assumption that talking about problems makes them go away. Actually, to believe this is to debase the differences between (the importance of) some talk over others. In this, and throughout the novel, you will feel Jake's humiliation as he exposes himself to successive therapists (and their patois), the sort of people who, outside wifely pressure, he wouldn't have walked up a wet step to say hello to.

Women

Towards the end of *Jake's Thing* Amis twists the knife in women as less able than men, academically, artistically, and the sense now is of a writer running on spite. His diatribe however is his way of exploring the false consciousness of psychotherapy, that is its point. One of Amis's biographers, Eric Jacobs (1995a: 315), said that when Amis's marriage to Elizabeth Jane Howard 'hit the rocks': 'love wore off, then liking, then sex, though not necessarily in that precise and orderly sequence'. Amis would have allowed them to go their separate ways but Mrs Amis wouldn't and so began the descent into 'counselling', 'feelings' and '*libeeedo*'. Initially, Amis and Howard consulted psychotherapists jointly, one of whom prescribed 'procedures' aimed at rejuvenating their physical love-life. Amis re-invents all of this in the persons of Jake and his fat wife Brenda and, in doing so, allows both himself (and us) to jeer at therapy. He especially sneers at Dr Rosenberg's advocacy of 'inceptive re-grouping', 'non-genital sensate focussing' and the use of the 'nocturnal mensurator', the latter a machine which, strapped to the penis, measures any and all activity that occurs as darkness falls. Jake (or is it Amis?) 'takes the mickey' out of this, lacerating the verbal shallowness (of psychotherapy), its formulaic, pseudo-scientific meanderings, its faux portentousness.

Yet Amis really tried to save his marriage, dutifully attending therapy sessions, suffering fools (un-gladly). His son Martin commented (2000: 308–9): 'What really impressed me is how much *boredom* [original italics] he put up with.' Amis's best bile was reserved for group therapists. Being 'in group' was fashionable at the time and although we can only guess at the make-up of its clientele one imagines there being ample scope for derision. Note the narrator's summing up of a group-work session: 'To limit the danger of cardiac arrest from indignation and incredulity Jake had made an agreement with himself not to look at his watch'. Reflecting further on his Dad's torment, Martin Amis was lost as to 'what sustained him', why he persevered with activities he found daft and soul destroying. Perhaps it was his dread at being left alone, especially indoors, at night. Not wanting to lose his night companion, he was prepared to put up with considerable aggravation to prevent this. One wonders at the number of couples who enter therapy at the behest of one of them, the other biting their tongue into two pieces at the humiliation of it all.

Of course Amis gained little from therapy and eventually tired of it. As Jacobs recounts, towards the end of 1979 he was complaining to his closest friend Philip Larkin about:

> a wife who puts herself first and the rest nowhere, and constantly goes out to GROUPS and WORKSHOPS [Amis despised the *word* workshop] and crappy 'new friends' and total loss of sex-drive. I haven't had a f*** for more than a year and a w*** for over a month. Don't tell anyone.
> (Leader, 2000: 876)

Don't *tell* anyone? Later on, he writes to Larkin: 'What a feast is awaiting chaps when we're both dead and our complete letters come out' (Leader, 2000: 479). As indeed they did.

Is that all there is?

No. *Jake's Thing* also tells us about how novels are written, how an intelligent imagination talks back to a phenomenon like psychotherapy within a culture of (perceived) diminishing scepticism and intelligent enquiry about matters in general or, as Amis puts it, a gullibility duped by the fashionable dodge of asserting that something can be explained simply by naming it. Today's dodge is that talking about it – whatever *it* might be – diminishes it, draws it out, soothes it, cures it. In an irreligious age the psychotherapists become a 'secular priesthood' (North, 1972), an ecclesia bestowing warmth as well as the reassurance that matters are never entirely your responsibility, that no one is at fault for anything, really. Prototypical of the 'age of counselling' is Dr Theodore Dalrymble's account of a male patient who dragged a girlfriend into an alleyway and brutally battered her: 'The thing is, doctor', said the patient, 'she was doin' me head in, know what I mean?' Or if you prefer: 'There were psychological reasons for doing what I did and please respect these.'

Reception

Although cherished by some, the male chauvinism of *Jake's Thing* led to its being vilified by many. It came out at a time when feminist critiques of literature and culture were robust and assertive and so most of the flack came from the belief that he was anti-women, that Jake was really a cipher for what Amis could never say *outside* of fiction. And yet Jake differs from Amis in important ways. Jake drinks only moderately whereas Amis swam in alcohol, *he wrote books about it*. Amis retained life-long friendships with people (not women) whereas Jake has few associates that he sees as worthwhile. More importantly, though, Jake is irritating, querulous, racist and snobbish: he has little time for others and self-satisfyingly so (Amis too was irritating and querulous, but not the other two). So that the novel's intrigue (and technique) is to set Jake up for contempt whilst managing, at the same time, to parody the world he is forced to inhabit as incrementally odious and believably so.

But supposing Jake's views *are* Amis's: that is, what if, in a general sense, a writer's beliefs are perceived as morally objectionable or out of kilter? Putting this slightly differently, should writers reflect the dominant mores and culture of their society? According to Alex Comfort (1948: 8) the 'correctness' of a writer's perspective, his/her degree of conformity to critics and audiences, has nothing to do with his stature as a writer and that there is, actually, a rich history of novels that scandalised society or, in the case of D.H. Lawrence's *Lady Chatterley's Lover*, provoked litigation as an instrument of suppression. In countries like Ireland or the former Soviet Union, more drastic action, including banning books or refusing visas to writers, were effective mechanisms of control. Russian novelist Boris Pasternak was prevented from receiving his Nobel Prize in this way and, in Ireland, James Joyce's *Ulysses* was prohibited reading for years.

Amis's take on the relationship between fiction and society was to attend to the writing itself. He believed that advice to read this or that writer because 'they were important' was misleading and he confessed to not knowing what such advice meant. Quoting the philosopher J.L. Austin, he remarked that: 'being important is not important' and, referring to the writer Elizabeth Taylor (Amis, 1992), Amis admiringly notes her disdain for literary criticism whether praiseworthy or otherwise. The contention is that what is said *in* novels is what matters, but not in any sense of playing to the galleries, vested interests or critics. Alvarez (2005) dates the 'myth of the artist' from about the sixties – the age of gurus – wherein the work and its writer become indistinguishable. He mentions especially Sylvia Plath whose suicide contributed significantly to her icon status. Conversely, her husband, Ted Hughes, was demonised as a vicious chauvinist, a conviction only overturned with the publication of Hughes's later poems. Curious, the numbers of intelligent American women willing to overlook Plath's bouts with depression before she had even met Hughes.

Howard's way

Elizabeth Jane Howard's endless recriminations and 'advice' resulted in Amis seeing her as the epitome of malevolence and he laces this hatred throughout *Jake's Thing*. Before moving on, however, let's peek into *her* memoirs (2002: 438):

> I thought that once we divorced ... we might become friends. I couldn't have been more wrong. He maintained an implacable resentment towards me for the rest of his life. He was painfully open about this, in interviews and in the two novels [including *Jake's Thing*] he wrote after I left. I found that very hard to endure because it wasn't how I felt and because he was intent on wiping out anything good that there'd been about the eighteen years we'd spent together.

Novels are fiction and fiction privileges itself above factual accuracy or historical truth. These are not its function albeit, occasionally, novels come before the courts charged with libel. But this is rare since there's always the fallback argument that they are make-believe, *stories*. However, that doesn't mean that novels are autobiography. The confusion comes about in that autobiography, whilst ostensibly true, often conveys nuances and 'between the lines' messages that suggest the creative impulse at work, what diarist Alan Clark (1992) termed being 'economical with the actualité': indeed as Amis says in his *Memoirs*, (1992: 306): 'Many times I have put into people's mouths approximations of what they said, what they might well have said, what they said at another time, and a few almost outright inventions.' Nevertheless, with biography and autobiography matters are approached from the outside in, from the general to the particular, from prior knowledge of, or interest, in its subject. The novel, alternatively, infers the universal, moving from the particular, in this instance Jake and Co., through narratives that inform our lives as we read them. Its structure becomes a springboard from which a writer, using the events of his life, jumps into make-believe and we, the readers, supply the rest.

An example of how this works comes from Amis's fear of travelling on the London Underground. This fear was explained to him (in real life) by Freudian psychiatrist Dr Gerald Wooster as a conflict arising from his (traumatic) birth. The explanation is reprised in the novel (1979: 247) when Jake, like Amis, an only child, tells a psychiatrist that what especially terrifies him is waiting in the underground for a train that will never come!

And, he said, me being afraid of nothing arriving in my underground was all to do with my mum being afraid of something arriving in her underground. Isn't that marvellous? Especially nothing being the same as something. I tell you, that cheered me up, it really reassured me. I thought, I may be a bit peculiar but at least I'm not as barmy as to come up with that.

Note the conjunction of 'something' with 'nothing', how Jake places intellectual superiority over a psychiatric profession that is depicted throughout the novel as stupid and incompetent. Amis, it should be said, did not disdain *all* psychiatry. Jim Durham, a friend of his, was 'a rare kind of fellow in several ways, not the least that of being about the only sane and sensible psychiatrist I have ever met' (Amis, 1992: 309). It was Durham who referred Amis to sexologist Dr Patricia Gillan who also comes off, surprisingly so, relatively unscathed in his writings. What Amis's ire seems to (eagerly) fix on are certain variants of the profession. Psychoanalysis of course with its queer interpretations and prodigious deployment of symbols. Here is Amis's view of it (1992: 117) in a nutshell:

Freudianism has probably been instrumental in fewer deaths than Nazism or Marxism, though it is surely one of the great pernicious doctrines of our century with its denial of free will and personal responsibility. But it is of course enormous fun, combining the discovery of curious information about people's inner selves with the clue-chasing, puzzle-solving pleasures of the old-fashioned detective story.

Next in line of disrepute are the sterile platitudes of 'the groupies' and their 'feel good' self-effacement, the personification of the 'beatlesque' mantra that 'all you need is love'. Amis's special bile for these had long toppled into a paranoia that an intelligent world had been overtaken by platitudes and cheap rhetoric. Last, come the rude mechanicals, the behaviourists, with their skin-deep techniques and crass assumption that life is an academy of maladaptive learning. For them, mental distress stems less from what happens in the womb, less the ability to form *deep and meaningful* relationships and more a failure of learning, of unwillingness to appreciate that logic is the basis of life generally. The latter practitioners have decided to place factual evidence and measurable, therapeutic outcomes as top of their agenda claiming significantly higher scores for these than other approaches. There are a range of incidentals that attend such claims but the point, often missed, is that therapeutic effectiveness doesn't necessarily lead to truth and success can be as dependent on false assumptions as anything else. We need to reward practicality but not overlook that power of theory and perspective to contribute to the sum total of experience within which the practice obtains or loses meaning.

Jake's wife

There are early indications of Brenda's disaffection with Jake, but it is only in chapter three that she really 'has a go'. Enraged at his rudeness to her friends, she rounds on him, flinging crockery at his head (though I suspect she deliberately misses). But whilst a marital referee might score this chapter even, look at how Jake's internal monologue governs the action, how the narrative allows him final adjudication about what has, and is, happening.

A particular quirk of Jake's is that he will often say what he doesn't want to, or only partly wants to and he notices this tendency in others. When Brenda (pp. 28–9) attacks him over his behaviour towards Mr and Mrs Mabbott he says he's sorry and will make sure he does better next time. But only some minutes earlier he had wanted to tell Brenda that the idea of those two having noticed anything in the least objectionable was a load of rubbish. It is this interior dialogue which provides direct access to Jake's thoughts, feelings and attitudes. What is voiced, out loud, alternatively, are stratagems on Jake's part intent on keeping the peace, minimising interpersonal friction; in fact, anything for a quiet life. How much this speaks for all of us is debatable but I suspect it does, a lot. If, for instance, one takes as 'read' that in psychoanalytic therapy the reliability of self-disclosure is low – unconscious resistance or avoidance playing its part – then where does this leave non-analytic therapies? Is there perhaps at work an unconscious by another name? Or, possibly, the unconscious takes a rest from therapies which it 'sees' as non-threatening? Or, in the novel's terms – and certainly in the couple and group therapies to which Amis was pressured into – we might adopt Jake's tactic of partial, deceptive or even non-disclosure. Either way, it becomes a 'toss-up' as to how much of the unconscious you allow into therapy. The unconscious is a bit like love, it happens to you and so you believe in it.

Another of Jake's irritants is that others don't (but *ought* to!) know things such as that Mexico is *not* in Latin America or that a revolution occurred in France in 1848 (p. 38). Here he is (pp. 156–7) savaging Dr. Rosenberg's ignorance, an action that deflects the impending terror of attending 'group' with its (too near the surface) emotions and its disaffection for things intellectual. This is Amis's favoured sore point, the 'touchy-feely' brigade's intolerance of intelligent understanding. 'Rosenberg didn't know where Freud functioned, what had happened in 1848, or who James Bond was … Rosenberg had never heard of the Titanic, Haggis, T.S. Eliot, Plutonium, Lent … Herodotus, Sauternes … Van Gogh, Sibelius, Pelota, Lemurs, … and Hadrian's Wall.'

Whilst this is defensive, Jake can also be aggressive and no more so than when belittling the *language* of therapy. See, for instance, the start of chapter six or watch his missile accuracy (p. 86) as he attacks Dr Rosenberg's psychobabble. At one point Rosenberg says to him: 'I meant your personal reaction in mental and emotional terms' and Jake replies: 'How I feel, you mean?'

Amis also arms Jake with decided views on persons of non-English origins. Dr Rosenberg bemuses Jake. I mean, how can this (improbable) Irishman conduct therapy at all or at least not without: 'rushing around the corner all the time to get a lot of strong drink inside him' (p. 91) and there are plenty more asides aimed at non-Englanders. But it is therapy which suffers the brunt of his firepower and *Jake's Thing* is crammed with barbs such as Jake calling Dr Rosenberg 'the scientist of mental phenomena' (p. 44) or one-liners about psychologists as 'students of the mind' (p. 115) or how even their appearances upset him. Meeting a certain Dr Cobb, 'a kind of highbrow marriage counsellor', Jake (1992: 118) can't avoid noticing his hat: 'which was of the round, rough, tufty sort affected by middle-class people in television series about village life, was enough to assure me that nothing of which I could make the slightest use was going to come out from under it.'

In effect, Jake is (as Amis was) caught up in a farcical situation over which there is little control: hence the venom, even the barely concealed racism against the Irishman with the odd name. Amis had once remarked to his son that he went along with the psychological hocus-pocus merely to 'show willing' to his wife. He was perhaps before his time, the kind of Englishman, notes Bradford (2001) for whom the involvement of other people in what was essentially a private problem was worse than the problem itself.

My own past

Something of this belongs to my own past. Distressed that my mother was seriously ill, I visited a psychologist who turned out to be of the behaviourist persuasion. I can't remember how she was dressed but she had sweaty hands and a melamine attaché case (slightly ajar) with bits of (electrical?) wire protruding from it. Wary of the attaché case, I didn't take to her much. In such situations, it's little things like this that matter, verbal nuances, noises off, nose-pimples. I mean, can a psychotherapist who wears socks *inside* sandals be taken seriously or one who sports a full-length caftan circa Woodstock 1969? Later on, with another 'therapist', I lost the will to go on when she exclaimed in nasal New Yorkese that she found the Lady Boys of Bangkok, appearing locally, 'really odd', a real puzzle.

Culture matters and tends to be under-discussed in psychotherapy circles because this would undermine those of its assumptions which bypass politico-economic but especially cultural-ethnic implications. Look at the exchanges (on p. 154 for example) to do with emotion and nonsense and note Jakes' sense of affronted *Englishness*. With Amis, as well as Jake, there is always the inference that 'psychological mumbo-jumbo' is a 'put-up job' by foreigners – including Americans.

I think aversion to therapy also comes from constructs of privacy. In England, people walk along public streets by and large to get from the supermarket to the DIY shop. On the Continent, alternatively, they may use the street to drink coffee or wine, stroll, meet, talk, argue or even foment revolutions. It's an issue of privacy. That 'An Englishman's home is his castle' doesn't merely affirm ownership, it's also about enclosing body and soul, a boundary whose role is to contain as well as withstand. Jeremy Paxman (1999: 118) notes how a word for privacy doesn't exist in French nor in Italian. In England, it is fundamental to any conception of social interaction. One recalls the mother of R.D. Laing, aghast at his choosing a branch of medicine where people discuss their private lives, 'hanging their dirty linen out to dry'. So that whilst it cannot be denied that 'the counselling professions' have held sway in England as much as anywhere else, they have not done so without critical dissention and an occasional certain moral distain.

Comic despair

Jake's Thing is a novel of comic despair with sinister overtones. It is self-centred and whiney about the fatuous inability of some, mainly women, to behave with intelligent sense. Although neither Amis (nor Jake) would have had little tolerance for existentialism – where is the *argument*? – neither would they have disagreed with Sartre's dictum: 'Hell is other people'. OK, so we have a novel of despair, anger, dissolution. Listen as Jake (pp. 21–2) talks back at himself:

> In that moment he saw the world in its true light, as a place where nothing had ever been any good and nothing of significance done: no art worth a second look, no philosophy of the slightest appositeness, no law but served the state, no history that gave an inkling of how it had been and what had happened. And no love, only egotism, infatuation and lust.

This was Amis's mindset when writing *Jake's Thing* and it disdains fulfilment or happiness in any form. Freudians would savour this massive projection on Amis's part, the loathing and despair properly belonging to his own psyche, the cynicisms and rages, the exasperated, if hidden, recognition of his failures and growing inadequacies both as writer and as a man. So too should we see the downward spiral of self-abuse incurred by his excessive drinking. However, for this one must believe in projection to begin with and Amis dismissed it as circular, one more insult to intelligence.

So what are we then left with? An angry ageing man, embittered by women, isolated from a fractured society and determined to pen novels of rage and loathing? No, because Amis was a wordsmith who never wrote a bad sentence and *Jake's Thing is* painfully funny in many places. Some of the set pieces, for example its final page, display a menacing brilliance that make you gasp. Yet the way he makes language hit its targets is precisely, provocatively, pleasurable. Note, for instance, the ongoing jibe (p. 62) against naming things as a form of explanation:

> Brenda: 'Comfort eating. What Dr Thing said I'd been going in for because of feeling sexually inadequate. Had you heard of it?' Jake replies: 'I think so, anyway it's clear enough what it's supposed to mean, which is all balls. If there's anybody who feels sexually inadequate it's me and I haven't started eating my head off. Just another example of thinking that if you name something you've explained it. Like ... permissive society.

Is this true do you think? What other instances of psychiatric theorising might warrant this criticism? Do you think that Amis's celebration of the 'stupidities' of the therapies is a tad excessive? One imagines them more vulnerable to criticism in the 1970s than now. In time, behaviourists would come to see their own tinkering as cumbersome and they quickly metamorphosed to cognitive therapy although never *quite* losing their 'simple equations' veneer.

And today? How would Amis's critique work against therapies today? Ironically, more comfortably than it did back then. The drive for evidence-based practice now forces a scepticism about therapies that don't 'show results' and this works hardest against the humanistic counsellors. And as for psychoanalysis, always deficient in the evidence stakes, it is now, in Britain, if not a spent force, then usable only in watered down, superficial forms.

And so, these days, Amis's dislike of sham and cant might make him a welcome bedfellow for psychologists who increasingly see what lies beyond cognitive behaviourism as only so much blather. But he would surely acknowledge the peculiarity of a Freudian psychology that led to Joyce, Hitchcock, Dali, Stravinsky and much more, compared to behavioural therapies that alleviate much human misery without adding much to what we know about being human.

Reputation

Amis's reputation follows him. Literary (Marxist) critic Terry Eagleton has labelled Amis: 'A racist, anti-Semitic boor, a drink-sodden, self-hating reviler of women, gays and liberals' (Henshaw, 2007). Eagleton, a man of sobriety and propriety, is surely confused? Does it matter that Amis, like many writers, drank alcohol, or was disappointed with life? That he was *not* anti-gay is amply demonstrated by his biographers (Jacobs, 1995a; Leader, 2006). To be enthusiastically heterosexual doesn't imply anything about the sexual orientation of others and besides, his friendship with Philip Larkin, sometimes reads like love. Was he anti-Semitic? Or racist? Probably not. According to Jacobs (1995a: 39) he relished differences of class and race:

> He could always laugh at a joke about an Englishman, a Scotsman and a Jew or about an earl or a dustman, so long as it was a good one. But his enjoyment came from the comic possibilities of the differences between them. He could not find funny a joke based on the stereotypical notion that Jews or earls were funny or ridiculous, let alone contemptible, just for being who they were.

However, he did speculate on the shortcomings of ethnic groups. We've mentioned Jake's glib comments about the Irish therapist who needed drink to keep going. Equally, though, did Amis surmise that 'the British philistine' could be 'crude, ignorant, aggressively uncultured'. Amis had once been sent a book by a Wilmot Robinson called *The Dispossessed* which claimed that Jews and liberals, combined, were edging white people out of power and influence in America. Reviewing the book he was initially sceptical, but he began to reflect:

> Hard on the Jews, natch, but then you pick up the Sunday paper and in *The Sunday Times Review* alone you find Susan Sontag, G. Steiner, a Russian-Jewish novelist, Freud, Steven Marcus, a new US Jewish pop novelist and no doubt others – yes, Mel Brooks – all writing or being written about, and you start shamefacedly and reservedly thinking that he may have something.
> (Jacobs, 1995a: 346)

The kindest interpretation is that these ruminations don't bear thinking about too much, they were little more than idle, half-hidden inklings. Yet he could have concealed these things more than he did. Also, there is something especially obnoxious in racism which expresses itself benignly as though it doesn't *really* matter, as if it's just a private game (often played out with pen pal Philip Larkin).

Yet it is possible to miss him:

> The bewildering thing is that, after having seen all his cussedness catalogued and inventoried – friends insulted, children ignored, wives betrayed, with maximum pain inflicted whenever possible – everyone on his side of the pond regards him with backhanded affection: wonderfully wicked, magnificently rude, hilariously horrible, and so on. The orneriness became ornamental.
> (Gopnik, 2007)

And sanity? therapy? cure? Amis took his hang-ups to the grave as he knew he would:

> Physical disease is treatable and curable; some mad people are also curable, chiefly by drugs, and if nobody seems to know how they work, who cares? But the poor old neurotic might just as well spend his money on booze and sex magazines. I have noticed that women rather like going to see shrinks whereas men tend not to. But then women are keener on going on holidays than men. Merely an observation.
> (Amis, 1992: 119)

A barbed observation, again floated publicly, but with a sting in its tail. Paraphrasing Freud: 'I take away the neurosis so that people can get on with the ordinary miseries of life' is all very well except that, for the neurotic, the distinction doesn't exist. The neuroses *are* the ordinary miseries blown out of proportion by the unwanted fears that attend them. And their nuisance value is that the neurotic knows that their meaning are logically silly.

Coda

Christopher Hitchens (2002: 53) plotted Amis's progress from left to right-wing by mapping it to levels of success: 'Kingsley Amis – extremely funny when still quite left-wing; still fantastically funny when joining right-wing; less funny and more dystopian as positions solidify; bitter ironist towards the end; elements of self-parody in closing.' *Jake's Thing* comprises the last two of these: solidifying bitterness, self-parody, and with a dollop of 'see if I care'; but he would return, close to his life's end, with *The Old Devils* which won the Booker Prize and a rekindled reputation as a humane and considered writer.

References

Alvarez, A (2005) The myth of the artist. In C Saunders & J Macnaughton (eds) *Madness and Creativity in Literature and Culture* (pp. 194–201). Basingstoke: Palgrave Macmillan.

Amis, K (1961) *Lucky Jim*. Harmondsworth: Penguin.

Amis, K (1979) *Jake's Thing*. Harmondsworth: Penguin.

Amis, K (1992) *Memoirs*. London: Penguin.

Amis, K (1994) *You Can't Do Both*. London: Hutchinson.

Amis, M (2000) *Experience*. London: Jonathan Cape.

Beckett, S (1986) *The London Times*. 10 April.

Bradford, R (2001) *Lucky Him*. London: Peter Owen.

Clark, A (1992) Testimony given at the Matrix Churchill trial at the Old Bailey. November.

Comfort, A (1948) *The Novel and Our Time*. London: Phoenix House.

Gopnik, A (2007) The old devil. *The New Yorker*: Book Review Section.

Henshaw, P (2007) Amis was neither a misogynist nor a homophobe. *The Independent*, 9 October.

Hitchens, C (2002) Between Waugh and Woodhouse: Comedy and conservatism. In Z Leader (ed) *On Modern British Fiction* (pp. 45–59). Oxford: Oxford University Press.

Howard, EJ (2002) *Slipstream: A memoir*. London: Pan.

Jacobs, E (1995a) *Kingsley Amis: A biography*. London: Hodder & Stoughton.

Jacobs, E (1995b) *The Spectator*, 28 October: 28.

Leader, Z (2000) *The Letters of Kingsley Amis*. London: HarperCollins.

Leader, Z (2006) *The Life of Kingsley Amis*. London: Jonathan Cape.

North, M (1972) *The Secular Priests*. London: George Allen & Unwin.

Paxman, J (1999) *The English: Portrait of a people*. Harmondsworth: Penguin.

Shakespeare, W (1967) *Macbeth*. Harmondsworth: Penguin.

RICHARD III

There is a pleasure sure,
In being mad, which none but madmen
Know!
(John Dryden, *The Spanish Friar*, Act I, sc ii)

The historical context

Shakespeare's audiences would have known of England's recent civil wars (1455 –1485) between the Houses of York and Lancaster (called the Wars of the Roses, white and red roses symbolising the two Houses respectively) which the House of York won, a victory that placed Richard's older brother on the throne as King Edward IV. Hence, Richard's opening lines:

Now is the winter of our discontent
Made glorious summer by this son of York
(Shakespeare, *Richard III*, Act I, sc i)

The King being the 'son of York' and the winter of discontent the aforesaid civil wars (note Richard's ability, from the first, to 'make play' with words). As the action unfolds, therefore, Yorkists rule the roost, but with Richard an aggrieved fourth in line of succession, his brother Clarence and two child princes (his nephews) in line before him.

According to historians, Shakespeare needed to tread carefully when setting these matters before audiences (the play was first performed for certain, in 1633, before Charles I and Queen Henrietta Maria). However, it was written during the Elizabethan age with the intention of pleasing the House of Tudor, which had succeeded Richard III. Unsurprisingly, Shakespeare depicts Richard as the embodiment of evil and inimical to stability and good government. For Shakespeare, political stability and order were important; he believed their maintenance required strong and just leadership. So does his play finish with a Tudor dynasty heralding a new and promising age.

Richard III is one of Shakespeare's less structured/layered works and beset with contradiction and implausibility, but it was (and remains) the most sensational account of despotic ambition yet written, a powerful indictment of the acquisition of power by someone seriously deficient in exercising it,

Mesmerised, we watch a maimed psychopath scuttle his way to the top and, less engrossed, the banality of his downward spiral into fear and destruction. With *Richard III*, Shakespeare significantly takes English drama into the realms of psychological characterisation. At the same time, it's a play that also bears witness to a Providence which ensures that evil will devour itself so that, by its end, moral as well as political order will be restored.

A word about the supernatural

Today (reputedly) we live in a material world where science explains all (or soon will) and where hobgoblins are but infantile fancies of the impressionable or immature. Yet recall the widespread success of *The Exorcist* (Friedkin, 1973) with reports of people screaming or even passing out whilst watching it. Nor is there any shortage of artefacts, literary or pictorial, of the occult and the gothic in our midst. High street bookshops, for example, devote lengthy shelves to these and a Hobbit obsession testifies to our need for the hyper-real. More recent still, *The Sixth Sense* (Night Shyamalan, 1999) achieved extraordinary popularity as one of a bunch of such films – remember *The Blair Witch Project* (Myrick & Sanchez, 1999)? Yet we might see these as petty diversions which, returning from a night at the cinema, are quickly forgotten. Well, possibly, albeit this could be motivated forgetting, repressing a dread that apprehends more than cool reason ever can.

Of course, in Shakespeare's day, devils were real enough, and believed entirely capable of manifesting an earthly presence. Many of Shakespeare's plays interlock with events such as violent storms which, at the time, were deemed unnatural in origin, portents of evil, harbingers of moral and dynastic disorder. Most ordinary folk saw good and evil explicitly so that as an audience they would have expected events to be shown in black and white. In his more mature plays, straightforward comparisons are less apparent but whilst *Richard III* is amongst the Bard's earliest, it's an adept exploration of interpersonal psychology nevertheless. At the same time, the supernatural is but thinly veiled so that the tension conveyed lies in an exposition of human motive but with an added tincture of otherworldly vice.

Morality

We need to understand the theatricality of this. Morality plays, a genre of the period, were wont to include a Vice character, a motif combined of traditional elements of fool and jester. Thus could the Vice manipulate 'others in the play whilst interacting, as though on another plane, with the audience' (Lull, 1999: 8). Spectators might revel in a Vice addressing them directly or demanding money as it circulated amongst them. This Vice aspect is pretty obvious in Laurence Olivier's (1955) film performance where the camera rarely takes 'its' eyes off him as he campily limps about beckoning audiences to share in his secrets and lies, winking knowingly, lasciviously, delivering rapid-fire, witty asides. Like a veritable Max Miller, Olivier motions audiences to come *inside* the action, to abandon the safety of distance from the stage, to become complicit in mischief making.

But although audiences (now as well as then) see Richard as inhabiting aspects of the Vice, they also recognise the depth of characterisation as it works through a narrative that encompasses (a) evil coming into the world, (b) evil triumphant, (c) evil playing itself out, and (d) evil vanquished on Bosworth Field. In other words, this is Shakespeare, and so Richard is no mere Vice. Imbued with complex and not easily ascertainable traits, he is 'the first of Shakespeare's tragic figures to emerge from the conventions of contemporary melodrama with a genuine force of personality' (Traversi, 1955: 181). Imagine you're in an Elizabethan audience – or even a contemporary one – aghast at this creepy character scamping about the stage, just about human, weaving verbal cobwebs of entrapment, without conscience.

> *Enter Richard, Duke of Gloucester*
> Now is the winter of our discontent
> Made glorious summer by this sun of York;
> And all the clouds that lour'd upon our house
> In the deep bosom of the ocean buried.
> Now are our brows bound with victorious wreaths;
> Our bruised arms hung up for monuments;
> Our stern alarums changed to merry meetings;
> Our dreadful marches to delightful measures.
> Grim-visag'd war hath smooth'd his wrinkled front;
> And now, – instead of mounting barbed steeds,
> To fright the souls of fearful adversaries, –
> He capers nimbly in a lady's chamber
> To the lascivious pleasing of a lute.
> But I, that am not shap'd for sportive tricks,
> Nor made to court an amorous looking-glass;
> I, that am rudely stamp'd and want lov's majesty
> To strut before a wanton ambling nymph;
> I, that am curtail'd of this fair proportion,
> Cheated of feature by dissembling nature,
> Deform'd, unfinish'd, sent before my time
> Into this breathing world, scarce half made up,
> And that so lamely and unfashionable
> That dogs bark at me, as I halt by them;
> Why, I, in this weak piping time of peace,
> Have no delight to pass away the time,

Unless to see my shadow in the sun
And descant on my own deformity;
And therefore, since I cannot prove a lover,
To entertain these fair well-spoken days,
I am determined to prove a villain,
And hate the idle pleasures of these days.
Plots have I laid, inductions dangerous,
By drunken prophecies, libels, and dreams,
To set my brother Clarence and the King
In deadly hate the one against the other:
And if King Edward be as true and just
As I am subtle, false, and treacherous,
This day should Clarence closely be mew'd up,
About a prophecy, which says, that G
Of Edward's heirs the murderer shall be.
Dive, thoughts, down to my soul: here Clarence comes.
    (Act I, sc i, 1–41)

Initial thoughts

In this soliloquy (soliloquy is talking without, or with disregard for, the presence
of hearers) Richard tells us what makes him tick. The lines are staccato-like but
they drip word-play and irony too, although not so as to lessen their credibility.
In the last line, when he says 'dive, thoughts ...', we might surmise that he's
been running these ideas (merely) through his head – not so – he *wants* to parade
(his) cleverness, chicanery, and treachery, itemising his deformities and the misery
they've brought him. He despairs that women spurn him and that even dogs in
the street bark as he passes: nature has sinisterly pushed him into an
uncomprehending world, ill equipped to proceed *except* by playing false, piping
others to heartbreak and death.

    Richard is a whizz at what we nowadays call role play. All things to all
people, he's the kind who tells you he's on your side whilst stabbing you in the
back. Moreover, nothing brings him regret. He luxuriates in other's difficulties:
watch when he bumps into his brother Clarence being taken to gaol, an
imprisonment that Richard has engineered. Not to worry, he tells Clarence, he,
Richard, will speak to the King, their brother, on his behalf. Moreover, he adds,
as the poor sod is led away: '... this deep disgrace in brotherhood touches me
deeper than you can imagine' (Act I, sc i, 111–12). Yeah, right. You might, at
this point, wonder why people can't resist his charms, see through his
manipulative ways. In essence this is due to his insight that people are *prone* to
flattery and persuasion. Further, he believes they get what they deserve. In this,
he is the prototype for W.C. Fields' dictum: 'Never give a sucker an even break.'
Like a rat, Richard pollutes everything around him and the effect is brilliantly

theatrical because exhibitionistic. It's as though Shakespeare has Richard 'send language out on a spree, ribald, dauntless and spoiling for a fight' (Tynan, cited in Smith, 1966: 7). At times this makes the lines sound improvised, as in Act III, sc iv, 59 when Richard, suddenly swapping guile for controlled venom, spews out his accusations as loaded questions:

> I pray you all, tell me what they deserve
> That do conspire my death with devilish plots
> Of damned witchcraft, and that have prevailed
> Upon my body with their hellish charm?
> > (Act III, sc iv, 58–61)

Insects

Taking a lead from Anne's description of Richard as 'any creeping venomed thing that lives', some actors have decked him out in non-human apparel. Famously, Laurence Olivier employed an avian image, the crow (John Lydon of the Sex Pistols would base his Johnny Rotten persona on Olivier's interpretation). More recently, Antony Sher released Richard as a spider, the actor bounding about the stage on tentacle-like crutches. Said New York Times critic Frank Rich (1985: 27):

> Sometimes Mr Sher deploys the crutches as if he were a manic pole-vaulter, leaping about the stage like a maimed, mutant grasshopper. The result is an uncommonly fearsome villain whose grotesque deeds and distorted physique are accompanied by an aura of sadomasochistic sexuality.

Yet while Richard is frequently depicted as an arachnid, less than human, he is also 'alive, he is himself alone, he is what part of ourselves would like to be, free from the censor conscience' (Eccles, 1964: xxii) and though Richard belittles himself – not for him the amorous antics of the bedroom – watch, nevertheless, as he seduces women. He *knows* that women fantasise about sex and that neither humped back nor twisted tongue need be a barrier to winning 'love'. Consider the literary tradition of 'Byronic Hero', a 'larger than life' figure, moody, intellectually superior, 'forced' into arrogance, abnormally sensitive, conceited, cruel. It comes from Lord Byron who was rumoured to be: 'mad, bad, and dangerous to know' and whose poetry gives the type its name. The Byronic Hero towers above those around him but is also haunted by memories that impel him to act morally correctly. In Bronte's (1847/1996) *Jane Eyre,* Mr Rochester exemplifies the type and although there's much that separates Rochester and Richard, the sexuality of 'the flawed protagonist' helps us comprehend Anne's 'conversion'. Together with Richard's opening soliloquy, you might now like to read Act I, sc ii where Richard courts Anne into marriage and death.

It exemplifies, I think, Richard's disdain for people except as ciphers for his cynical capers and fatuous giggling. In a Manhattan performance (by Christopher McCann):

> Richard ... capers towards his end, unfettered by conscience or moral restraint. Equally nimble of mind, tongue and affect, he rollicks about, tugging his leather-braced knee with a chain on his withered arm, and loving up the audience with piping voice and the seductive glint of a sweet nihilistic fool.
> (London, 1998: 64)

The scene with Richard and Anne is about deformity, sexuality and reparation. In Ian McKellen's version, a jackbooted Richard dances his way through the action, his left arm dead, his right otherwise engaged. At one point he takes a ring from his finger with his teeth replacing it on Anne's marriage finger. Why does she permit this, an act as fully erotic as it is of marital implications? Just what *is* it about him that turns her on? It reminds me of a story about Greta Garbo who had just watched Jean Cocteau's (1946) film *Beauty and the Beast* and how, at the end, with the demise of the beast, Beauty duly wins her handsome Prince (think Brad Pitt) only for Garbo to murmur, with what Lee Siegel (2005) called a 'slow, silky pout', 'Give me back my beast!'

The psychology of getting one's own back

Here is Freud's take on Richard's opening soliloquy:

> the bitterness and minuteness with which Richard has depicted his deformity make their full effect, and we clearly perceive the fellow feeling which compels our sympathy even with a villain like him. What the soliloquy thus means is: nature has done me a grievous wrong in denying me the beauty of form which wins human love. Life owes me reparation for this, and I will see that I get it. I may do wrong myself, since wrong has been done to me.
> (cited in Clemen, 1968: 7)

This is standard psychoanalytic fare, an interpretation of compensation in the classic style of: 'I will transform self-loathing into violent sexuality towards others, especially women.' Several of the play's elements support this view, for example the emphasis on childhood and remembrances of things past. When, for instance, Richard's mother speaks of her relationship with her infant son, this too spews from projection. Here it is:

> Thou cam'st on earth to make the earth my hell.
> A grievous burden was thy birth to me;
> Tetchy and wayward was thy infancy;

The school-days frightful, desp'rate, wild, and furious;
The prime of manhood daring, bold, and venturous;
Thy age confirm'd, proud, subtle, sly, and bloody:
More mild, but yet more harmful, kind in hatred.
　　(Act IV, sc iv, 167–73)

Contemporary readings, notably Antony Sher's (1985), incorporate projection as well as sibling rivalry, displacement and compensation. Equally, though, could these lines imply that Richard was a 'bad egg' from day one and with little need of maternal neglect. Sher's psychoanalytic usage, the bad mother projecting her deficiencies into the son, is packed with theatrical possibilities, but it begs the question, central to concepts of madness, of the relative contributions of nature and nurture.

　　Neither does psychoanalysis exhaust psychology's ability to describe, possibly even explain, what's going on. A behaviourist explanation, for instance, might depict King Richard as a product of maladaptive learning, his conduct comprised of automatic responses to scapegoating and blaming. Equally, he has clearly discovered the rewards that vice brings. We may suppose that his mother's 'blaming' is of long standing and his self-mocking does suggest emotional infantilism, the internalisation of 'the matriarch' a clue to his campy, sniggering sexuality. Whether or will, and despite one's pet theories, the push nowadays is to appraise Richard's character psychologically, the psychology that most artists prefer being psychoanalysis. However, that such appraisals sufficiently account for literary creations becomes doubtful because the moment evil assumes its place, earthly psychology loses pace. Evildoing raises the question of free will, whether we choose to do wrong or are driven to it by maladaptive learning, genetic inheritance or a Freudian unconscious (see Chapter 3). Richard never doubts *his* power to choose as he rasps on about peace being weakness and how he determines to do his worst, come what may. Do we take this at face value? Is he worthy of such self-assurance? Can certainty make things true? Do any of us have free will?

Tempting Anne

To some, Richard's wooing of Anne invites derision, it's so far-fetched. For others, fascination ensues as, predator like, he ensnares and bags her. He has told us that women are not for him. As if. The fact is, this is what he wants us to believe and of course he attracts women, even when (as in Anne's case) the circumstances are manifestly unpropitious. So what's he on about when he denies that he can be a lover? Perhaps his disclaimers reflect denial. Or is this him again cynically mollifying the effects of his actions, skewing the perceptions others may have of him?

　　A difficulty with *Richard III* being an early work is that its psychological technique is comparatively weak, its characters not fully worked out in human terms. Instead we see an ambiguous Richard, in part metaphysical, a devil metaphor, that needs stamping out before it disrupts nature (i.e. England). But, as Ian Johnston (2007) notes, other aspects of Richard's humanity are also on show. (See also Hammond's (1981: 97–119) rebuttal of Richard as one-dimensional). For instance, he is very droll, his pleasure in laying verbal traps for people whilst *telling us about it* gives him great fun! He delights in macabre self-effacement, so that he informs us (absurdly) that even the dogs bark: '...as I halt by them'. But, we may ask, *why* halt by them? Is he revelling in deformity, harbouring satisfaction in his predicament? That might explain the time spent in pulling Anne, which is that he takes pleasure in humiliation, being spat at. When she wishes her spit was poison, he replies: 'Never came poison from so sweet a place' (Act I, sc ii, 147).

Such speculations may be too quick though and it's tempting to decipher matters in overtly sexual ways when less speculative approaches might do. Also, Richard's is a well-practised cynicism that constantly undercuts how others see him, leaving them wondering always about what he is up to.

Women, feminism and Richard III

The Anne scene is long and, you might think, implausible. Some have seen Anne as willing victim and so undeserving of sympathy. For me, she is a kind of 'straight man' to Richard's music hall 'turn'. So that, when playing on her widow's grief he stunningly announces that it was he that murdered her husband, one expects her to bugger off stage left. But she doesn't. Curiously, she remains, subjecting herself to a master class in male verbal dexterity. Notice Richard's use of words (such as 'love') when talking to, at and around her. Remember too that this is a *play* – one doesn't just bring logic to it, emotional 'senses' inform what happens between them (and us). And, as well, Shakespeare's audiences would have stood close to the action, reality in osmosis with illusion, Anne's curses literally reigning down on them.

Anne's capitulation *is* difficult to comprehend. Its understanding lies ultimately in playgoers' willingness to suspend their finer judgement. Time and again, Anne rebuffs Richard with language that would petrify Dracula. But he works on her like a sculptor and Shakespeare has blessed him with deep intuition, the cleverest lines and good opportunities for dramatic effect. Note his intimation that *she* is responsible for Henry's death, that it was love of her that made him kill her husband. Such warbling causes her to fear and loathe him so that when he invites her to stab him she loses it. For although wanting him dead, 'when push becomes shove' she can't insert the blade. And when she utters: 'I would I knew thy heart' it's a wary resignation that yet prevents her caving in. When Richard bids her to wish him farewell she replies: 'Tis more than you deserve; / But since you teach me how to flatter you, / Imagine I have said farewell already' (Act I, sc ii, 224–5).

Generations of theatregoers have puzzled over the successful wooing of Anne. I mean Richard can hardly believe it himself. Relishing his newly acquired 'lover' status, he chats to himself (and us): what a 'wondrously handsome man I now must be! They'll need a dozen tailors to drape me for I'll outshine any mirror!' This is rubbish. He knows it wasn't good looks that won fair Anne and so do we.

He has become, says Anne, her 'teacher' but in what sense? In *Macbeth* (this volume, Chapter 9) we will examine whether reason governs actions, whether right and wrong are distinguishable and if it is possible to do wrong knowing it to be such. For example, how does reason become secondary to desire or need? Anne ought to know better in her dealings with Richard and not allow passion, the lesser part (of us), to determine her reactions but she doesn't, collapsing into subservience.

Sex and power

Nina Burleigh (1998), an American author, well respected, a White House correspondent, married, recalls meeting Bill Clinton, en route to a funeral no less. Having noticed the President sexually eying her up, she says:

> There was a time when the hormones of indignant feminism raged in my veins. An open gaze like that, at least from a man of lesser stature, would have annoyed me. But that evening I had the opposite reaction. I felt incandescent. It was riveting to know that the President had appreciated my legs, scarred as they were. It took several hours ... to shake the intoxicated state in which I had been quite willing to let myself be ravished by the President, should he have but asked. What is it in some of us, that *powerful men* [my italics] make us pliant and willing with a mere glance?

So too does Richard attribute 'victory' over Anne to 'dissembling looks', his, that is, but with not a little collusion on her part such that thoughts and emotions become unable to fight free of each other. Hark back to Ms Burleigh's references to 'intoxication', 'riveted' and 'power'.

The mind boggles at how the President would have handled alleged 'wrongdoing' with Ms Burleigh: in respect of Ms Lewinski he had said, with clipped enunciation and much finger wagging (Clinton, 1998):

> But I want to say one thing to the American people. I want you to listen to me. I'm not going to say this again. I did not have sexual relations with that woman, Miss Lewinski. I never told anybody to lie, not a single time, never. These allegations are false. And I need to go back to work for the American people.

Dismissively, he shoos all accusations away: 'how dare you', he seems to say, 'how *dare* you allege these things'. Now compare this to Richard's opening soliloquy, in particular at how both Richard and the President construct their sentences. Watch the President's superb use of 'I' and examine this same tactic when, about halfway through, Richard suddenly switches from 'our' to 'I'. Later, when allegations of sexual relations (with Ms Lewinski) became unanswerable, it transpired that everything rested on what was *meant* by 'sexual relations'. Mr Clinton *had* had a sexual relationship with Ms Lewinsky but had not had sexual relations (that is, intercourse). In this he acted immorally. Nevertheless, his was a brilliant distillation of words and intonation. Like the veritable mackerel in the moonlight, he shone *and* stank at the same time.

Moral equivocation

Apart from some nightmarish doubts near the end, Richard too shows little moral rectitude, submerging most things in equivocation. In *Richard III* everybody ducks and dives, watches their backs, tries to stay out of trouble. Equivocation is at its most telling at the Tower of London when Brackenbury, the Tower's lieutenant, is handed a writ requesting he surrender Clarence. Suspecting mischief, he wriggles out of it thus:

> I am, in this, commanded to deliver
> The noble Duke of Clarence to your hands.
> I will not reason what is meant hereby,
> Because I will be guiltless of the meaning.
>   (Act I, sc iv, 91–4)

A case of 'turning a blind eye' if ever there was one. It is a theme that will re-emerge with greater force in the case of the Macbeths (this volume, Chapter 9).

Contemporary usage

Richard dominates the play. Whenever he exits stage left or right, we can't wait for his return. We *like* watching this cripple overcoming obstacles even when playing the scoundrel to do so. Yet is he also a displacement object, someone to whom we project darker, baser, instincts. Ian McKellen's interpretation bears this out where he argues that its importance rests not on 'Great Drama' status but on its continued relevance. Locating the action within Hitlerian despotism may be to expose the allure of the fascist impulse, at least for some. Others may find such renderings one dimensional, a 'literalisation of what even Richard recognises as improbable [and which] flattens the story into sheer and unrelenting grimness'(Coursen, cited in Jackson, 2000: 104).

Fascist expansionism, in McKellen's version, fits the political aggression of the Tudor period where, under Henry VIII (and Cardinal Wolsey), England exercised a pan-European influence integral to its evolution as a unified, unifying State. At a conscious, theatre-going level this works well especially for those of us reluctant to question the clandestine and primitive nature of our motives. We strive to keep the better sides of ourselves in control and much that we desire, we keep in check. Appraising the goings on of Richard, personal and imperial, the appeal to mythical power, black-shirted arrogance, ethnic superiority, sexual superciliousness and sadism, why do many of us react with concealed glee?

Poetic justice

As the drama closes, the protagonists, Richard and Richmond, display nervous apprehension' and calm assurance in turn. Whilst Richmond sleeps the sleep of the just, poor Richard is beset by nightmares. *Poor* Richard? Are you starting to feel sorry for him too? At this point (imminent war) he is pricked momentarily by conscience, but resolved to fight on. But how real is this? Is it a ruse to win our sympathy, to play on our charitable impulses? Psychopaths reputedly are expert at this, manipulating other's fears and hopes, enticing goodwill with false promises only to dash it coldly and without regard.

There is a saying: 'mad, bad or just plain sad' that summarises the psychiatric diagnosis of 'psychopath', particularly its indissoluble combination of immorality and insanity. Contemporary psychology disregards notions of 'bad' since it lacks utility in treating offenders. This however raises the question of whether psychiatry's disregard of morality is workable in the wider sphere of responsibility towards others.

In *Richard III*, evil is characterised as the devil and Richard is often referred to as such: 'With odd old ends stol'n forth of holy writ, And seem a saint when most I play the devil'(Act I, sc iii, 337–8). This is the declaration of someone who known no bounds, earthly or spiritual, someone who hates his fellow man (But, 'Alack, I love myself' (Act V, sc iii, 188). He is an accomplished hypocrite, brutal, vicious, egocentric, cruel, unnatural, conceited, blasphemous, the perfect anti-Christ. Yet he becomes King and dares call himself 'The Lord's Anointed.' Knowing no conscience he is, says Jan Kott (1967: 45) 'beyond cruelty: beyond psychology; he has no face'. Although he is given a visage by the actor, even when it is of a buffoon, it remains 'the highest form of contempt: absolute contempt.' He possesses, as well, that most frightening of psychopathic elements, unpredictability. For example, Hastings thinks he knows Richard's position on public affairs and so blunders into Richard's accusations of treason with the remark: *if they have done these things*: Richard pounces: 'If! Thou protector of this damned strumpet, Talk'st to me of Ifs? Thou are a traitor: Off with his head!' (Act III, sc iv, 73–5).

It's a play about death and its absurdity except at the end when absurdity is bartered for fear. Because when it's Richard's time to die, the chicanery stops.

Soon he will be butchered like a pig. From the head of the corpse the crown will be torn. A new young king will now talk of peace, forgiveness, justice. And suddenly he gives a crowing sound like Richard's and, for a second, the same sort of grimace twists his face. The face of the new king is radiant again.

(Kott, 1967: 46)

The poet Patrick Kavanagh once cautioned: 'the self is but an illustration'. Tempus fugit. Kings, governments come and go and that which is believed fundamental alters. So are we to bear witness to our lives not just in Rogerian 'here and now' terms but in lieu of the cultural values to which we give testimony but which enable us to make life becoming for all, not just ourselves. One of the lessons of *Richard III* is that self-aggrandisement brings disaster, that usurping the values, wishes and feelings of others is to be defended against. It warns against psychologies that (a) preach the merits of emotional wilfulness whilst neglecting an ethics of reason and (b) ignore how oppressive political systems impinge on individuals rendering them psychologically impotent. Richard is destroyed because of his desire to dominate *at any cost*. As such, he loses sight of how much he has left himself open to annihilation. Our current prioritisation of 'the self' also risks the unethical that echoes the invariable narcissism that lies at its heart. One of the 'prophets' of our age, Michel Foucault (1982: 210) has stated: 'Shall we try reason? To my mind, nothing could be more futile.' Constructs, born of emotion, are more liable to fashionable fancy: how easily have we become 'passion's slaves' in the flight into selfhood.

Films

Three interpretations of *Richard III* are available on DVD. There is the Laurence Olivier version (1955) which remained the yardstick performance for years. Another is Ian McKellen's (Loncraine, 1996) interpretation which is in so many ways different. A third, by Al Pacino (1996), takes the play through rehearsal and out on to the streets where the actors discuss it with passers-by.

Watching these performances 'back to back' will afford insights into the tension between theatricality and realism. Olivier's treatment is wonderfully theatrical as he spits out Shakespeare's text with tongue-whip efficiency. He is bitterly sly, crow-looking, *devilish* though not the devil, but sufficiently so that he can *play* the fool to (as he sees it) actual fools.

McKellen's Richard is less playful. Set in the 1930s, during the rise of militarist dictatorships in Europe (and with rumours that some English Royals were not averse to fascism) the film has a realist veneer in that the evil stems from human disposition and political despotism. The emphasis is less on the origins of evil and more about how evil 'succeeds' as political ambition. In all cases, of course, Richard's ascendancy rests on weaknesses in others, their inability to confront him outside his frames of reference. We've mentioned that complicity plays its part in Richard's machinations. Coming into contact with him mesmerises people into responding in ways that suit *him*. This has its exception with some of the women characters, in Act IV, sc iv for instance, largely because these women operate outside the main action of the play.

All three films underwrite the play's openness to interpretation. Interpretation, however, can involve radical shifts in time, gender, location and so on. Some believe that rendering Shakespeare in contemporary terms should be the first port of call. Others see the relevance of Shakespeare embedded within the language of the plays. Todd London (1998: 24), artistic director of New York's New Dramatists, reflecting on contemporary productions commented:

> Increasingly ... his plays seem to me like someone else's dreams, dreams about which I can be eternally curious and only momentarily connected. They may be the most extravagant, beautiful dreams ever placed on stage but ... they remain remote. Seeing the plays had its satisfactions, but only reading them slaked my thirst.

One further point. Do not be surprised, watching these films, at the discrepancies from the printed texts as we now have them. Shakespeare's plays are long and few productions proceed without cutting or telescoping the material.

References

Bronte, C (1996) *Jane Eyre*. London: Smith, Elder. [Original work published in 1847]

Burleigh, N (1998) King of Hearts. *Mirabella*, July.

Clemen, W (1968) *A Commentary on Shakespeare's Richard III*. London: Methuen.

Clinton, W (1998) White House News Conference, January 26, 1998. Available from www.washngtonpost.com/wp-srv/politics/special/clinton/stories/whatclintonsaid.htm

Cocteau, J (1946) *Beauty and the Beast* [film]. Paris: Lopert Pictures.

Coursen, HR (2000) Filming Shakespeare's history: Three films of Richard III. In R Jackson (ed) *The Cambridge Companion to Shakespeare on Film* (pp. 99–116). Cambridge: Cambridge University Press.

Eccles, M (1964) *Richard III*. New York: Signet Books.

Foucault, M (1982) Afterword: The subject and power. In HL Dreyfus & P Rabinon (eds) *Michael Foucault: Beyond structuralism and hermeneutics* (pp. 208–26). Chicago: University of Chicago Press.

Friedkin, W (1973) *The Exorcist*. Hollywood: Warner Bros.

Hammond, A (1981) *Richard III*. London: The Arden Shakespeare.

Johnston, I (2007) Personal communication.

Kott, J (1967) *Shakespeare: Our contemporary* (2nd edn). London: Methuen.

Loncraine, R (1996) *Richard III*. Hollywood: MGM/UA.

London, T (1998) Shakespeare in a strange land. *American Theatre,15* (6), 22–5, 63–6.

Lull, J (1999) *King Richard III*. Cambridge: Cambridge University Press.

Myrick, D & Sanchez, E (1999) *The Blair Witch Project*. Hollywood: Haxan Films.

Night Shyamalan, M (1999) *The Sixth Sense*. Hollywood: Spyglass Pictures.

Olivier, L (1955) *Richard III*. London: London Films.

Pacino, A (1996) *Looking for Richard*. Hollywood: Fox/Searchlight Pictures.

Rich, F (1985) Stage: London quartet of Shakespeare royalty. *The New York Times*. 26 June, 27.

Shakespeare, W (1964) *Richard III*. New York: Signet Classics.

Sher, A (1985) *Year of the King*. London: Chatto.

Siegel, L (2005) Down the tube: Sexy beast. *The New Republic*. 31 August. Available online at: *http://www.tnr.com/*

Smith, G (1966) Critic Kenneth Tynan has mellowed but is still England's stingingest gadfly. *The New York Times*, 9 January, 7.

Traversi, D (1955) Shakespeare: The young dramatist. In B Ford (ed) *The Age of Shakespeare* (pp. 179–200). Harmondsworth: Penguin Books.

CHAPTER 6

THE YELLOW WALLPAPER

A dame that knows the ropes isn't likely
to get tied up.
   (Mae West)

To begin

This is a disturbing book whose effects are not diminished by brevity and were
it a thousand pages long, it would still be difficult to put down such is its terror.
It's a story of someone going mad as told in the happening of it. You are invited
to 'listen in' to a nameless, bedridden woman as she develops a fascination with
the yellow wallpaper in her room and how this paper acts as a reflector of the
demons in her mind. Although a novel, the book is autobiographical in tone,
Gilman having experienced several bouts of depression in her own life. It is
also an (early) example of a patient contesting a psychiatric diagnosis by
providing an alternative framework for her problems. Thus is this novel a
foundation text that reconstructs the nature of mental illness and the ownership
of medical knowledge.

    Written in the first person *The Yellow Wallpaper* takes the form, loosely, of
a diary which is kept secret from the narrator's husband, John, a doctor, who has
confined his wife to an upstairs bedroom – previously a nursery – whose seclusion
is effected via bars on the windows and a gate running across the stairs.
Noticeably, she is attentive to his instructions whilst his tone towards her is
patronising, if seemingly warm. Indeed, his loving demeanour cloaks that
patriarchal desire to eclipse any female behaviour that smacks of non-compliance.
In other words, there is 'a woman's place' which, clearly, the neurotic violates
by definition. The novel's doctor-husband combination brilliantly satirises a
medical dominance that essentially masquerades as caring and paternal. Time
and again Dr John addresses his wife gently and affectionately but which belies
his subversive control. She is his 'little goose', his 'little girl', brim full of 'silly
fancies', a delicate flower. But flowers must be nurtured, left to their own devices
they wither and die. The message is this: women in distress need male expertise
to put them right, women who question this merely confirm their
unreasonableness as well as unreasoning natures.

The book

Let's trace this lie through the book. 'John laughs at me', she says, 'but one expects that in marriage.' To begin with, she is forced to distinguish between reason and emotion in respect of her gender and although she claims to suffer, she also accepts her husband's denial of the reasons for her pain. As far as John is concerned, her complaints are 'one thing after another, give way to one and another will take its place'. Actually, his demand that she act from reason whilst, at the same time, treating her as infantile smacks of 'Double Bind Theory' (Bateson et al. 1956) (see next chapter, p. 82) and we can see how this works to demean her. Even her occasional anger is, she feels, unreasonable and she strains to stay in control 'before him, at least': 'He says that no one but myself can help me out of it, that I must use my will and self-control and not let any silly fancies run away with me' (Gilman, 1981: 22).

The wallpaper

Initially the paper challenges her aesthetic values: 'I never saw a worse paper in my life: one of those sprawling flamboyant patterns committing every artistic sin' (Gilman, 1981: 13). Very quickly however her aesthetic distaste turns to disgust resulting in a series of epithets: 'repellent', 'revolting', 'unclean yellow', 'lurid orange', 'sickly sulphur tint'. Apparently she complains to John about the paper's oppressiveness but he simply laughs, telling her that giving way to such fancies will hardly help her improve. And besides, he says, think of the cost of replacing it! And then the paper starts looking at her as if it knows something. Its patterns turn into crawling images with unblinking eyes, bearing hallmarks of sinister threat. 'I can see a strange, provoking, formless sort of figure, that seems to skulk about and behind that silly and conspicuous front design (Gilman, 1981: 18).

This is the child's tendency to illusion but coupled with an adult perception that 'the reality' is 'silly', the selfsame epithet her husband uses on her. She too recalls that children are prone to illusions – misperceptions based on something real – and a staging point of the novel is when illusion becomes delusion – misperception not based on anything at all. There are signs that she still controls her faculties regardless of what John says, for example she wants to get away. But then, slowly, the paper begins to take over. 'You think you have mastered it, but just as you get well underway in following, it turns a back summersault and there you are. It slaps you in the face, knocks you down, and tramples upon you' (Gilman, 1981: 25).

According to Barbara Hochman (2002: 91):

> Her efforts to follow the pattern are repeatedly frustrated, but her desire to do so is a recurrent – in fact, a pervasive emphasis in the story. She is preoccupied

with the design's 'lack of sequence' and bent upon resolving the seemingly irrational pattern into a sort of mimetic representation – one with a beginning, a middle, and an end.

Therefore, in absorbing the paper's sensuous malevolence, she seeks to minimise its manipulation of her psyche, to rearrange its pattern jigsaw-like into a manageable whole. But she is aware she is getting worse, and on a particular night wakes John telling him that she's not gaining weight and wants out of the room. And his reply? '"Bless her little heart," said he, with a big hug, "she shall be as sick as she pleases! But now lets improve the shining hours by going to sleep, and talk about it in the morning"' (Gilman, 1981: 24).

As time passes she jealously believes that he is looking at *her* paper and this makes her fear him. The paper now smells, the stench infecting the whole house. Horrified, seeing her husband's 'kindnesses' for what they (really) are, she locks herself in and begins to crawl about the floor, much as 'the women' in the wallpaper do. Creeping this way and that she will suddenly turn so as to catch sight, through her window, of women creeping outside. Except, who or what are these women? Perhaps this is an example of Doppelgänger syndrome (see this volume, Chapter 10) where it's her self that she sees 'swaying off in the open country, creeping as fast as a cloud shadow in a high wind'. Actually, later she will say that she did indeed come from the wallpaper like the others who now creep around so fast.

Interpretation

As with Kafka's *Metamorphosis* (this volume, Chapter 7) innumerable interpretations have been pulled from Gilman's novel. We know that her doctor has warned against intellectual activity, especially the deleterious effects of reading, and that her husband agrees with this. And it is stimuli starvation that causes her to detect movement in the wallpaper, eventually seeing figures, including herself, crawling within and behind it. In a way, she 'reads' the wallpaper as a means of self-revelation. The paper envelopes her, its graphic yellowness perturbs and challenges her. She and the paper play a war game, the battlefields comprised of repressed sexuality, powerlessness and madness.

Female sexuality was both a repressed and suppressed commodity at the time, its physical expression very much a function of male demand, and women could be seriously ignorant of sexual matters. (Marie Stopes 1880–1958, for example, a pioneer of women's rights, claimed that only after visiting a doctor, did she realise her marriage was unconsummated.)

It took exceptional courage to confront male ascendancy and few women possessed the emotional, political or economic wherewithal to even try. Even if successful (typically with the assistance of a sympathetic – and wealthy – husband) a price still needed to be paid for economic or political advancement. Especially since its reissue as a Virago Classic (1981), *The Yellow Wallpaper*

71

has served as an important women's rights document. Showalter (1985: 142) calls it a 'haunting and passionate protest [and] a modern feminist classic, a paradigmatic text for how critics and historians look at the relation between sex roles, madness, and creativity'. It extends understandings of madness by symbolically treating the heroine's troubles less as a 'condition' and more as clusters of reactions embedded within social proprieties, especially marital roles.

Feminism

For that reason, many women have seen *The Yellow Wallpaper* not only as a story of illness but as a flagship opposition to any social order that refuses women the vote or self-sufficiency and, above all, that fears (female) creative imagination. In light of Gilman's 'rationale' for writing the book, a feminist ambition, few would deny Quawas' (2006: 38) summation:

> The wallpaper ... clearly represents not only the narrator's own divided self but all women who are bound and inhibited by a society that insists that women are childlike and incapable of self-actualisation. *The Yellow Wallpaper* depicts insanity in relation to sexual politics and states that madness is connected to the female social condition.

In Gilman's time, women came second to men as per social custom. She, however, was a feminist, a socialist and political activist. An author of non-fiction as well as fiction, *The Yellow Wallpaper* is her acknowledged masterpiece, its depiction of incipient madness a barely veiled declaration of resilience and protest. Gilman had married at age 24, apparently for love, but with misgivings about what wifely duties normatively entailed. So did she saddle herself with a conflict of freedom of thought versus the rules of domesticity. It was this which led, in 1886, to a mental breakdown and consequent meeting with Dr S. Weir Mitchell, *the* leading psychiatrist of the day and whose sub-speciality was the rich and famous. (Among his wealthy, and intellectual, patrons were the novelist Edith Wharton and the poet Winifred Howells.)

Gothic

Gothic fiction covers a wide spectrum but essentially its action will take place in a castle or other timeworn place. It will have a graveyard perhaps, or crypts, and the hint of things not fully controlled by natural phenomena. Ironically it was the coming of rationalism, specifically the emergence of 'science', which heightened the sense of the unnatural and/or gruesome as in, for instance, Mary Shelley's *Frankenstein* (1818). Electricity, for instance, in addition to giving off light, was imbued with life-giving powers, a mix-and-match monster shocked into existence by the harnessed voltage of lightening.

The Yellow Wallpaper has a gothic style, its story unfolding within 'ancestral halls' in which a distraught female is terrorised by a superior male imbued with scientific know-how. Confined to a room, Gilman's character, perhaps conscious of being tainted by a 'female heredity', turns it into a space wherein, dreamlike, that which is real, isn't, and vice versa. And so she builds her fantasy, splitting her intolerable anxiety into the relative safety of the pathological collage that lines the walls and from which, it seems, there is no escape. Like Gregor Samsa (this volume, Chapter 7) the room siphons off her humanity leaving her in an altered status, a derangement, that makes things bearable if just momentarily. For Gregor, there was never going to be much hope: here, a rebirth of sorts will take place but to what end? The room used to be a nursery. Did something awful happen there, possibly related to the heredity she mentions at the novel's beginning? Her one gladness about being in the room is that it spares her daughter the apprehension of threat that continues to reside within it.

The sinuous lines and oscillating abstractions of the sulphurous yellow of the wallpaper torment her (Showalter, 1985: 141)

This is because yellow signifies everything that is unrecognisable, threatening, foreign. The motif of 'the postcolonial' brings contentiousness to a fiction otherwise contained within feminist and psychiatric remits. As we noted in Chapter 2, the postcolonial necessarily implies political intent in the writing of a novel. Some have read into *The Yellow Wallpaper* motives of cultural and even racial superiority. According to Roth (2001: 145):

> The tale is haunted by an Oriental fantasy [that is, the orientalism of the wallpaper] and this functions as an environment or surround for the dominant American subjectivity represented by the narrator of this tale. There is no question about the oriental identity of the art: Gilman calls it 'florid arabesque', and since she trained briefly at the Rhode Island School of Design, she would have known what the term implied. Domestic ornament in the 19th century contained sign systems that articulated a complex of attitudes about the imaginary East.

Gilman does depict the wallpaper as an extreme irritant. Likening it to toadstools, she declares that it smells horribly: 'The colour is repellent, almost revolting; a smouldering unclean yellow, strangely faded by the slow-turning sunlight ... a sickly sulphur tint' (Gilman, 1981: 13).

If this seems far-fetched it's worth noting that, at the time, patterned yellow wallpaper within fiction is often described in distasteful and/or objectionable terms. Throughout the history of art, be it music, architecture or literature, the 'arabesque' (elaborate and repeated geometric forms), although admired in the

West by some, was depicted as inferior to Western art forms. In addition, the use of particular wallpapers was contemporaneously a bone of contention amongst interior decorators both artistically and hygienically. Doctors, for instance, 'criticised wallpaper as part of their battle against neurasthenia. (Indeed) the exasperating effect of patterned wallpaper on invalids was a medical commonplace of Gilman's time' (Roth, 2001: 146). Gilman *is* intriguing to read in this context. In another of her novels, *Herland* (1915/1979), elements of racism are detectable where the superior females, who inhabit the story, are depicted as Aryan. Critics divide on the significance of *Herland* but it supports the status of *The Yellow Wallpaper* as an imperial tract of sorts. The only problem is that weighting this thesis against feminist interpretations requires an ingenuity of understanding that feminist accounts don't, and Gilman was very much a feminist.

Nevertheless Susan Lanser (1989) notes how a feminist 'ownership' of *The Yellow Wallpaper* crystallised through the lenses of white-skinned and middle-class female writers. She argues that, amongst the nineteenth-century elite, the term *yellow* denoted Chinese, Japanese, Poles, Jews, Italians and Irish with an extension into disease, ugliness, inferiority and decay. In this way, the wallpaper links to a political consciousness whose true fear is alien 'culture', unease at a 'superior' white culture succumbing to the yellowness of 'the other'. It is this supposed supremacy which renders art universal, supposed because it sees Western art as the peak of creativity. Thus do 'write back' novels, such as *A Question of Power* (this volume, Chapter 12) provide a rhetoric of regional pride whilst celebrating a newer universality derived from racial and ethnic sub-groups that are non-Aryan. The complicatedness of this is perhaps unwelcome where clear-cut pairings of individuals with pathology, be it psychological or physical, renders matters more accessible to professionals whilst justifying their interventions. Yet if feminism, gender, economics and oppression can explicate madness why not cosmic/racial forces that arguably inhabit a collective unconscious that unites individuals through history, myth and imagination?

Psychiatrists

In the nineteenth century, psychiatrists were inclined to bundle any and all non-conformist behaviour (of women) under the heading 'neurasthenia' otherwise known as 'exhaustion of the nerves'. A new diagnosis, it called for a new cure, and Dr Weir Mitchell just happened to have one. His very own concoction, he wasn't joking when he called it the 'rest cure' since it involved separation from immediate family and surroundings, total confinement to bed, overfeeding – obesity increased energy levels – massage, either by hand or electrics, all followed by a return to family life and its silent desperations. In Gilman's case, Weir Mitchell specifically forbade *all* intellectual activity which really was asking the impossible although she endeavoured to follow his advice, a decision that brought her even closer to the brink of madness.

These were the experiences she put into *The Yellow Wallpaper* (including the redoubtable Dr Weir Mitchell) and, in doing so, fashioned a book that revealed, as has none since, the relationship of madness to sociality and especially its loci of power instituted in medical and gendered constructs.

So why did she write it?

In *Why I wrote 'The Yellow Wallpaper'* (1913) Gilman states:

> For many years I suffered from a severe and continuous nervous breakdown tending to melancholia – and beyond. During about the third year of this trouble I went, in devout faith and some faint stir of hope, to a noted specialist in nervous diseases, the best known in the country. This wise man put me to bed and applied the rest cure, to which a still-good physique responded so promptly that he concluded there was nothing much the matter with me, and sent me home with solemn advice to 'live as domestic a life as far as possible,' to, 'but two hours intellectual life a day,' and, 'never to touch pen, brush, or pencil again' as long as I lived.

Unlike her unnamed protagonist, Gilman didn't have hallucinations and this may have afforded her greater leeway in asserting that the rest cure did her more harm than good. The cure's recipients may well have construed it as a punishment, its provisions representing *in extremis* the strictures that were the lot of middle-class married women.

In essence, women needed to demonstrate four qualities of 'good' womanhood: 'piety, purity, submissiveness and domesticity'. Failure to accede to these rendered them vulnerable to remonstration and, if need be, coercion. And if embracing 'good' matrimonial qualities opened avenues of self-aggrandisement, deference was still required both initially and as ongoing proof of marriage as fulfilment. Women might 'rule the roost' in the home in terms of housekeeping if not economic management but it was the male who foraged and earned, who exerted command within (and over) the extended world of the house and all its facets.

But Charlotte Perkins Gilman stepped outside domesticity, personally and politically, so as to make herself heard in the wider world. Ahead of her time, she fronted herself as author, socialist, economist, feminist, and although our interest is in her fiction, this too challenged assumptions about academic, economic and marital thought and their impact on the aetiology of female madness. At the time, in American literature, males occupied centre stage as fiction writers as well as being its major protagonists, Women, alternatively, either wrote romantic fiction or, within fiction, occupied the subsidiary position of walk-on part, incidental to the main action. Gilman changed that, *The Yellow Wallpaper* being central to her project.

By showing women rebelling against the dominant feminine ideal in Victorian culture, the fiction of Gilman broke with a nineteenth-century literary tradition that essentially upheld domestic ideology and tended to present female characters as either pious angels or shameful objects of pity and scorn.

(Quawas, 2006: 41)

Women, men and war

In 1869, responding to uncertainties between illnesses of organic, as opposed to psychological, origins, George Beard invented neurasthenia, identifying 'exhaustion of the nerves' as its origin. This exhaustion was believed due to the kinds of stresses endured by (a) the intelligentsia and (b) the upper classes. It takes little working out to see that this combination excluded 'the masses' as less eligible for consideration just indeed as Freud had done for *his* invention, psychoanalysis. But neurasthenia became especially a designer diagnosis tailored to women though not exclusively so. In *Regeneration* (Chapter 3), as we've seen, almost all the officers at Craiglockhart were diagnosed with it as were, over the years, a fair number of the 'great and the good' in the male population, psychologist William James, writer Gustav Flaubert and US President Theodore Roosevelt being examples. In sum, as many as ten per cent of late nineteenth and early twentieth century males were said to be neurasthenic. In the main though, it struck at females or, at any rate, females were the main recipients of its diagnosis and in the public mind it came to be seen as characteristic of 'the female state'.

It will help to examine this from the vantage point of one of its victims. Florence Nightingale's (1820–1910) chief biographer (Woodham-Smith, 1950) named her 'The Greatest Victorian of Them All' and she is remembered (with increasing dissention) as the founder of modern nursing. A brilliant statistician and administrator, she allegedly transformed the lives of British soldiers at war and was a moving force in reorganising late nineteenth-century British hospitals.

Returning from the Crimean War (1853–1856) where she had toiled ceaselessly at the Scutari Military Hospital, she exhibited symptoms of weakness, headache, loss of appetite, tachycardia, breathlessness and chest pain. Today, psychiatrists would probably opt for 'panic attack', 'stress', 'chronic fatigue syndrome' or 'chronic anxiety disorder' as likely explanations for these symptoms, with chronic fatigue syndrome the diagnosis of choice.

In a fascinating essay, Young (1995) notes how Nightingale's symptoms occurred in acute episodes, and that this suggested that she had contracted the infection chronic brucellosis. Nightingale had certainly caught fever at the Crimea but believed it to be typhus (Baly, 1996). Young concedes that her 'clinical picture' might fit a psychological description but asks why such a 'precise, energetic and inquiring woman' should succumb to invalidity so quickly and without apparent scientific explanation. Responding to this, Monica Baly (1996:

1040) allows that fever played its part, but also asks: 'Why did she stay in bed, or on a couch, for twenty years? The short answer [to which Young concurs in part] is that this was the treatment prescribed and that she acquiesced.'

In this, says Baly, she achieved much by way of secondary gain, using 'illness' to force changes in army and welfare reform as in expansion of poor law provision. That these reforms would have happened anyway is likely. What's clear, however, is that Nightingale knowingly embraced debility, embodied a 'condition' enshrined in social beliefs about inherent weaknesses in women and that this furthered her interests. Of course, Florence was famous and extraordinarily well connected inside government and even royal circles. Less prominent, less celebrated, personages were not so well defended and therefore likely to receive more robust treatment. These were women who, if:

> not locked up for falling victim to melancholy ... or moral insanity were at risk of neurasthenia, a mirror image of rebellion in which their nervous depletion was explained as the result of their incursion into the masculine sphere of intellectual labour.
> (Harrison, 2008)

Therefore diagnoses of neurasthenia curtailed behaviour believed to flout social convention even if, attempting to reify their identity, some women colluded with this in part. A variation on this is David Schuster's (2005: 700) assertion – as relevant now as before – that neurasthenia was a medical construction that allowed patients to 'personalise' their suffering, reinterpreting it in line with self-perceptions of their social position and obligations, *à la* Nightingale. That Gilman didn't 'get on' with Weir Mitchell is instructive in light of Schuster's comments, which is to say that whatever she forfeited as his patient she retained sufficient mental autonomy to critique his medical standing. Taking issue with his treatment, she redefined her tribulations as iatrogenic and in furtherance of a feminist agenda.

The treatment of neurasthenia

posed a problem. Matters were complicated by the prevalence of male patients since it just didn't seem the thing to prescribe 'rest cures' for *them*. Elaine Showalter (1985) comments on the movie *City Slickers* (Underwood, 1991) to show how American males were advised to 'recharge the batteries', in this instance by riding into the Wild West where men 'walk tall' and 'ride high' in the saddle. Whilst *City Slickers* was played for comedy, its darker side was explored in John Boorman's *Deliverance* (1972) where down-rapids canoeists, cut adrift from civilisation, encounter devils in human form. Their macho pretentions peeled back, their heterosexuality violated, they revolt into violence, destroy their devils, before scuttling back to the banalities of everyday living

They have been tested in ways they didn't expect, at least not consciously so, and not found wanting, in ways they also didn't expect.

For women, alternatively, rest cures were seen as eminently suitable, partly because it was assumed that they would docilely accept whatever restrictions were imposed. In addition to physical and mental rest – literal confinement to bed for months – the overfeeding led to weight gains of 40 to 50 pounds. It was a cure that demanded a forceful physician. Showalter (1985: 139) quotes Weir Mitchell on this point:

> When they are bidden to stay in bed a month, and neither to read, write, nor sew, and have one nurse – who is not a relative – then rest becomes for some women a rather bitter medicine, and they are glad enough to accept the order to rise and go about when the doctor issues a mandate which has become pleasantly welcome and eagerly looked for.

One imagines that if they weren't swooning before the Great Man entered the room they soon would be! Appignanesi (2008: 121) relates that Weir Mitchell once coaxed a lady from her bed by announcing that he would undress and climb in beside her if she didn't move. She relented at the sight of his underwear. Whether or not true, it uncovers the melodrama surrounding both the 'illness' and the omnipotent spirit of 'the cure'.

Reviewing Weir Mitchell's treatment of Amelia Mason, Schuster (2005: 706) notes her description of him as 'autocratic' and 'impersonal' but that she thought this made him a perfect receptacle for women's problems and secrets. Mason trusted him and had faith in his cure, which no doubt led to her having a positive outcome. Of course, a patient's trust (or distrust, or hatred, or whatever) in a therapist invites the question of whether the concept of transference adds to the meaning of what passes between them. When Mason tells Schuster that: 'A woman confides to a trusted physician what she could say to no other friend', in what way has the physician become someone else? We know that therapeutic effectiveness has something to do with a therapist's personality (whatever the technique involved). So Weir Mitchell may have provided 'character strength' to women otherwise 'disenfranchised' by marriage, in effect a male ego in which they could invest secrets, fears and desires. Without question 'the cure' was the 'counselling' of its time, becoming, in turn, the 'social boast' that 'being in therapy' can be today. In the United States, private clinics mushroomed and the 'well-to-do' flocked to them from across the world until, as ever, American influence spread, and the treatment was grabbed at by an impressed and welcoming Europe.

Of course, like newfangled treatments then and now, its supposed causative (physical/biological) nature would quickly evaporate. This is a process that normally follows someone's perception that the instrument of recovery is not a particular treatment or intervention but human involvement. In the case of the rest cure it was the inordinate attention given (to these patients) that really mattered, the intense medical, nursing and patriarchal attention. It is worthwhile looking at this because it holds true for many of psychiatry's other 'seminal breakthroughs'. 'Until his dying day Manfred Sakel (1959) insisted that insulin coma therapy cured schizophrenia. Sakel put patients into a deep coma before gradually bringing them out of it and declared astonishing results (as high as 80 per cent recovery rates) that were excitedly accepted by the psychiatric community. The following illustrative account is from a psychiatrist working at Coventry Mental Hospital around 1937:

> This 1,400 bed hospital … has a staff of six physicians all under 35 and all keen. [The hospital employed a full time pharmacist and (thank God in the writer's view) no psychologist.] Our trust is not in extra staff but in drugs … and now of course insulin shock is giving us a chemical procedure for the other great biogenic group [schizophrenia]. How the heart of the druggist has been gladdened these past four years!
> (Shorter, 1997: 211)

This is the Eureka phenomenon, an all-too-common occurrence in psychiatry wherein 'the magic bullet' is at last found, that there is now a way forward that is definitive, clear and incontrovertible. For rest cure, so too with insulin coma therapy and, as well, with Prozac and cognitive behaviour therapy (CBT). The professional's coma arrived when psychiatrist Harold Bourne published 'The insulin myth' (1953), a paper which dealt Sakel's treatment, unchallenged for thirty years, a death blow. Bourne stated (p. 964) that: 'there was no sound basis for the general opinion … that insulin coma therapy counteracts the schizophrenic process in some specific manner.' Bourne had noticed that as the treatment began, the intense interest generated a lot of drama due to the risks involved. However, repeated application overtook drama and with waning enthusiasm, success rates correspondingly dropped. Bourne (1953, 1958) had convincingly shown that whatever had 'cured' the patients, it wasn't the insulin. He later opined (1953: 964) that what insulin therapy *had* done, as with the rest cure, was 'provide a personal approach to the schizophrenic, suitably disguised as a physical treatment so as to slip past the prejudices of the age'.

Orthodox psychiatry rejected Bourne's analysis and it was only the arrival of substitutes, particularly chlorpromazine, that caused insulin therapy to decline. No doubt, as Bourne also ruefully observed, the 'philosophy': 'it can't do any harm to give it a try' drove much of the application of insulin therapy but it was a false dawn, and dangerous, for both patients and keepers. In retrospect, and given that some patients died from it, one wishes that those involved had acted more judiciously. But, it seems, psychiatric reverence for physical treatments prevails largely in line with the belief that, ultimately, mental illness will be reducible to biochemistry.

Who makes history?

Those who write it. History is also written *now,* with psychiatric history not an exception. It also reflects its writer's beliefs. For instance, in his *History of Psychiatry* (1997) Edward Shorter puts an (all too typical) spin on the treatments of nineteenth-century doctors. He doesn't mention *The Yellow Wallpaper* although we know that Dr Weir Mitchell read it, having been sent a copy by Gilman, and that he subsequently changed his mind about the efficacy of rest cures (see Showalter, 1985: 138–41). What Shorter's account seeks to do is define 'rest therapy' as a poultice for human troubles, a well-intentioned effort by a profession whose confidence was growing. Allowing some truth to this, Weir Mitchell is more recognisably an enforcer of acquiescence *disguised* as treatment. And to assert, as standard psychiatric texts do, that doctors were acting consistent with the social, political and sexual mores of their age, is to reify the charge that psychiatry follows fashion and is not the objective entity it claims to be.

Denying Gilman a voice was a first step in rejecting complementary approaches to understanding mental distress and its origins and it's something that continues to this day. One of the objectives of 1960s radical psychiatry was to counter this, drawing from non-medical intellectual traditions and disciplines. For example, merging literary criticism and orthodox historical methods forges narratives that integrate psychiatry into broader cultural constructs that can include patients' voices. This matters because discussions about aetiology, history and treatments of mental illnesses are only partial when owned by experts. Significantly, Louise Pembroke, a well-known psychiatric service user, resigned from the National Institute for Health and Clinical Excellence (NICE) objecting to the disproportional weight allotted to professional/medical advice (James, 2003). The question raised by this is two-fold: to what extent should non-experts become involved in the provision of care and, in a psychiatric context, should user participation be enshrined in law and not, as now, operate at the relative whim of healthcare providers and/or dedicated individuals?

Contemporary relevance

It is commonplace these days to relegate R.D. Laing – radical anti-psychiatrist of the late 1960s – to the psychiatric dustbin of history (Clarke, 2004). He is especially pilloried for having argued that families induce schizophrenia in their young less as a process of genetic transmission but more from skewed and oppressive family dynamics. Just as nineteenth-century psychiatry dictated that neurasthenia had a physical basis so is it currently asserted, with evidence from non-invasive brain scans, that schizophrenia is biologically driven. Nonetheless, within a context of female sexuality and psychosis, both contemporarily and historically, Laing's ideas take on indicative meaning.

The point is less about his claims concerning psychosis as that his provision of a vocabulary (of considerable technicality) equipped women as emancipators within psychiatric discourse. For many women, Laingian ideas became an expository method by which to amplify their concerns whether in fiction or elsewhere. Of course, *The Yellow Wallpaper* lives in its own time but Laingian thought adds both lineage and predictive weight to the political, gendered, motives of therapeutic activity. It remains indispensable in the exegesis of female-male dimensions both theoretically and practically in mental health care generally. One only has to turn to contemporary accounts of female mental distress (Millett, 2000, Johnstone, 2000, Appignanesi, 2008) to realise that women are still demonised through psychological processes that refuse to acknowledge male-female differentials as more than demographic statistics and not as experiences grounded in histories of oppression, of conditioning and an expectation of compliance.

The Yellow Wallpaper depicts a woman who chooses to inspect her own psychology within contexts of culture: social, marital, medical. This has involved a journey into madness, echoes of which are later found in Mary Barnes's (Barnes & Berke, 1991) account of 'going down', of regressing to an infantile state as a means of beginning anew. One imagines this as akin to collapsing a picture to its base elements before jigsaw-like reassembling it as a coherent whole. Rather than giving way to the wallpaper, allowing it to assimilate and possess her, she retains an ability to think *beside* her hallucinations. And if her collapsed husband continues to obstruct her path she will crawl over and away from him. On the final page she states:

> I've got out at last, said I, in spite of you and Jane. And I've pulled off most of the paper, so you can't put me back! Now why should that man have fainted? But he did, and right across my path by the wall, so that I have to creep over him every time!

The issue hasn't been about confinement to a room as much as the wallpaper's representation of the meaning of woman's place within oppressive structures. The giddy, childlike, quality of her liberty is the joy of starting over again.

References

Appignanesi, L (2008) *Mad, Bad and Sad.* London: Virago.

Baly, M (1996) Letters: Florence Nightingale's fever. *British Medical Journal, 312,* 1040, 20 April.

Barnes, M & Berke, J (1991) *Two Accounts of a Journey Through Madness.* London: Free Association Books.

Bateson, G, Jackson, DD, Haley, J & Weakland, J (1956) Towards a theory of schizophrenia. *Behavioral Science, 1,* 256–64.

Boorman, J (1972) *Deliverance* [film]. Hollywood: Warner Brothers.

Bourne, H (1953) The insulin myth. *The Lancet, 2,* 964.

Bourne, H (1958) Insulin coma in decline. *American Journal of Psychiatry, 114,* 1015–17.

Clarke, L (2004) *The Time of the Therapeutic Communities.* London: Jessica Kingsley.

Gilman, CP (1913) Why I wrote 'The Yellow Wallpaper'. *The Forerunner.* October.

Gilman, CP (1979) *Herland.* London: The Women's Press. [Original work published 1915]

Gilman, CP (1981) *The Yellow Wallpaper.* London: Virago. [Original work published 1899]

Harrison, K (2008) Diagnosis: Female. *The New York Times.* Available online at: http://www.nytimes.com/2008/04/27/books/review/Harrison-t.html

Hochman, B (2002) The reading habit and 'The Yellow Wallpaper'. *American Literature, 74*(1), 89–110.

James, A (2003) A disparity of esteem. *Openmind, 119,* 13.

Johnstone, L (2000) *Uses and Abuses of Psychiatry.* London: Routledge.

Lanser, SS (1989) Feminist criticism: 'The Yellow Wallpaper' and the politics of colour in America. *Feminist Studies, 15,* 415–42.

Millett, K (2000) *The Looney-Bin Trip.* Chicago: University of Illinois Press.

Quawas, R (2006) A new woman's journey into insanity: Descent and return in 'The Yellow Wallpaper'. *Journal of the Australasian Universities Modern Language Association, 105,* 35–54.

Roth, M (2001) Gilman's arabesque wallpaper. *Mosaic: A Journal for the Interdisciplinary Study of Literature, 34*(4), 145–62.

Sakel, M (1959) *Schizophrenia.* London: Peter Owen.

Schuster, DG (2005) Personalizing illness and modernity: S Weir Mitchell, literary women, and neurasthenia, 1870–1914. *Bulletin of the History of Medicine, 79* (4), 695–722.

Shelley, MW (1818) *Frankenstein.* London: Harding, Mavor & Jines.

Shorter, E (1997) *A History of Psychiatry.* Chichester: Wiley.

Showalter, E (1985) *The Female Malady.* New York: Pantheon.

Underwood, R (1991) *City Slickers* [film]. Hollywood: Castle Rock Entertainment.

Woodham-Smith, C (1950) *Florence Nightingale.* London: Constable.

Young, DAB (1995) Florence Nightingale's fever. *British Medical Journal, 311,* 1711–14.

A MOST HUMOURLESS SOLEMNITY?
METAMORPHOSIS

As Gregor Samsa awoke one morning from uneasy dreams he found himself
transformed in his bed into a gigantic insect.
(Kafka, 1999: 1)

Kafka disliked literary embellishments, excessive turns of phrase. His was a
detached inspection of emotions and he admired this in other writers as well. To
further this point I combine two observations from Vladimir Nabokov (1980:
256) and Malcolm Pasley (1963: 16) respectively: 'Kafka liked to draw his
terms from the language of law and science, giving them a kind of ironic
precision, with no intrusion of the author's private sentiments.' It is this which
provides:

> the probing intellectual element. This attempt to reveal what is positive by a
> process of negation has misled many critics into calling him a nihilist. Nothing
> could be more wrong. His object is to unmask: what he intends to lay bare is
> not a nullity but an essential core of truth.

His creation of an insect is not just artistic wizardry designed to impress. It's
about exposing inhuman propensities so as to better recognise and understand
them. It moves from section one to two in the space of a day whilst, between
sections two to three, the time frame is imprecise: parts one and two conclude
with violence and part three in death. The story is bizarre with things coming
into view procedurally, fitted around Gregor, jigsaw-like, his efforts to cope
also proceeding step by step. At first, Gregor little realises what's happening
but he quickly develops a sense of others treating him differently. For example,
whereas initially his food is carefully chosen and his room cleaned (by his sister
Greta) over time his space becomes a dumping ground, his sister losing interest.
Inevitably, actually at her instigation, he ceases to be referred to as 'he',
becoming, instead, 'it', a *thing*, dreaded, despised.

Like most of Kafka's 'victims', Gregor hasn't done anything to warrant his
altered state. True, he's had troubled dreams of late which might be due to guilt
or self-recrimination. On the other hand, guilt springs eternal, not just from a
troubled conscience but from anxiety in which is split off a 'self' that would
otherwise be repressed. It is well described by psychiatrist R.D. Laing (1960:
80–1):

> If the whole of the individual's being cannot be defended, the individual retracts his lines of defence until he withdraws within a central citadel, but the tragic paradox is that the more the self is defended in this way, the more it is destroyed. The ... destruction of the self in schizophrenic conditions is accomplished not by external attacks from the enemy (actual or supposed) but by the devastation caused by the inner defensive manoeuvres themselves.

We saw (this volume, Chapter 10) an anti-hero whose choices rendered him unknown to the better self that he wanted to be. States Jan Kott (1967: 75): 'Macbeth recognises that his existence is apparent rather than real, because he does not want to admit that the world he lives in is irrevocable. This world is to him a nightmare.' Wanting the nightmare to end, he wills it continue with more and yet more killing. He anticipates that the dead will lie in their graves but they won't, and in a hair-raising scene, General Banquo, whose death Macbeth orchestrated, appears before him, a projection of his guilt – perhaps – or, if you like, a supernatural visitation. And as for the world around Macbeth? His external world? Well ... he just about sums that up when he declares that: '... nothing is But what is not', perhaps literature's most striking instance of derealisation.

These are topsy-turvy worlds, selves turned inside out, manifesting in everyday life as delusion and self-deception. If what isn't is, then Gregor too may be living a nightmare, something from which he (and we) might escape. This is short-circuited however by a narrative that proceeds in fine detail spooling itself out as actual occurrences. Yet if not a nightmare, in what sense can an insect be taken seriously, as having human wants, needs, desires? It may be that Kafka violates the natural order so as to cut into new, if idiosyncratic, meanings and interpretations. Like the Laingian schizophrenic, faced with the threat of 'reality', Gregor orders his psyche into an internalised, safer, realm. For us, the question has always been whether such reconstructions qualitatively separate the 'schizophrenic's world' from the main, and if so, in what way? Is being Gregor, or schizophrenic, just another way of being human? Or is it to experience the world as trans-human? In his paper: 'What is it like to be a Bat?' Thomas Nagel confidently asserts that bats experience things. They do, of course, but only insofar as they 'perceive' their surroundings via sonar and with brains designed to deal with this. As such, to come into contact with an 'excited' bat in an enclosed space is to: 'know what it is to encounter a fundamentally *alien* [original italics] form of life' (Nagel, 1974: 438).

We cannot, therefore, know what this experience is like. If we try to imagine what it is to hang from a ceiling, to possess, like Gregor, the ability to crawl up and down walls, this tells us only what it might be like for *us* to be like that. What we really need to know is what it is like *for a bat* to be a bat.

Even if I could by gradual degrees be transformed into a bat, nothing in my

present constitution enables me to imagine what the experiences of such a future stage of myself thus metamorphosed would be like.
(Nagel, 1974: 439)

That the subjective experience of another organism is unknowable prevents us from really knowing what Gregor thinks or feels. And even if we allowed our imaginations to run riot we still couldn't explain what it is that prevents Gregor from screaming. You would think that waking up as a bug would strike a person with horror or destroy him/her with fear. But not a bit of it! In *Metamorphosis* things go on as before, as if nothing has happened. Why?

Is change as good as a rest?

Possibly: now that Gregor is an insect, 'he' can no longer imagine (or remember) what being human is like, the bat scenario in reverse. Yet why is he still preoccupied with getting to work on time? A bug concerned not to annoy his boss, what's that about? Is it conceivable that the whole thing is a joke on Kafka's part, a literary confidence trick, a tease? Perhaps George is insane, hallucinating his body, projecting paranoid delusions on to his family and employers? But what if he has always seen himself as insignificant, pygmy-like, second rate? What if his imagination has led him to reconstruct his family as a theatre of the absurd, a playground in which he tests the limits of their tolerance of, and depth of emotion for, him? Or, is his newfound status a satiation of masochistic desire, dependent, slurping up slops, pain, punishment?

On wakening, the first thing Gregor looks at is a cut-out he has attached to his bedroom wall, a picture of a woman in furs, her fleece-shrouded arm stretching towards him. Later when his sister and mother try to remove his furniture to give him more space he becomes so alarmed that he crawls to the picture and covers it with his body: the picture feels so comfortingly cold against his hot belly that rather than hand it over: 'He would rather fly in Greta's face' (p. 33).

The classic text on masochism is *Venus in Furs* (von Sacher-Masoch, 2006) and the allusion is hardly coincidental. Fed like an animal, experiencing humiliation, forced to cower, Gregor cowers with gratitude. In terms of insanity *and* masochism ponder these two things: von Sacher-Masoch's favourite 'slave name' when being punished by his mistress was Gregor and when asked his opinion on a pictorial cover for *Metamorphosis* Kafka suggested a man lying dejectedly across a bed. That is, the physical metamorphosis is entomological but the psychological anguish is human.

What can it mean?

Gregor's dehumanism signals (the archetypical) 'debasement of the individual' within the industrialised, corporate, faceless, state and this has been *the* commonest interpretation of *Metamorphosis*. For instance Kuna (1974: 51) has said that: 'The main aspects of economic man debased to a functional role ... emerged in Kafka's story in paradigmatic fashion.' Gregor complains about the demands of his job. Unable to enjoy a life of reasonable freedom, his existence revolves around alarm clocks, rushing to catch trains, irregular meals, meaningless travel. Today, people talk a lot about life-work balance and 'health and safety' regulations may effect differences to working practices. It's a fact, however, that individuals are still crushed by corporate muscle, for instance, the cancellation (and even theft) of pension funds and where capital no longer concerns itself with the retirement welfare of its people but of how to escape what they now see as an onerous responsibility.

Whilst this reading of *Metamorphosis* retains solid support it hasn't prevented other, different, interpretations. All schools of thought: literary, Marxist, Freudian, feminist, sociological, spiritual, existentialist, postmodernist, psychopathological, gothic, surrealist, have tried to fathom Gregor's predicament. Like the Steppenwolf (this volume, Chapter 10) his existence challenges what is not easily recognised or understood in conventional terms. With Harry Haller, a symbiotic relationship of man and beast has Harry reject the pretensions of bourgeois life whilst lapping up its luxuries, a reflection of the irresolvable dilemma of the relationship of individual to society. Within psychiatry, this dilemma coheres around schizophrenia and attempted solutions are presented along two fronts. Firstly, a genetic-biological flaw induces schizophrenia, the individual anatomically flawed from birth – before birth if you think about it – but with the metamorphosis to psychosis not erupting until early adulthood. It's a perspective laden with categorising, confining, stigmatising, separating. You might have thought that the recent closures of mental hospitals, with psychiatry repositioning itself as a community service, would entail a shift in ideology or conceptual attitude, but it doesn't. Community psychiatry doesn't necessarily lessen any commitment to psychopharmacology or custodialism, both now constituting a spreading therapeutic bureaucratisation with its 'at-risk registers', case-load management and proliferating, localised, secure units, motels of dangerousness and disaffection.

A second configuration is to see schizophrenia as an outcome of social – specifically family – influences. For example, Bateson's (Bateson et al., 1956) *Double Bind Theory* convinced some British psychiatrists (Laing, 1960; Cooper, 1972) that schizophrenic experiences were contingent on family persecution in which was posited a concept of 'elected victim'. This is where a family member disposes himself to being 'picked on', shrinking into tangles of (family) recrimination, judgement, abuse. In his classic tract on schizophrenia *The Divided Self* (1960: 82) R.D. Laing quotes Kafka thus: 'You can hold yourself back from the sufferings of the world, this is something you are free to do and is in accord with our nature, but perhaps precisely this holding back is the only suffering that you might be able to avoid.'

Concisely expressed, this is still the stuff of paradox, and paradox derails interpretation, ambiguity its primary hallmark. Kafka depicts the fantastic as 'real' and his combining of concrete terms and elliptical content is not unlike psychotic language where ideas are at once comprehensible yet unworldly, the unworldliness residing in the association of ideas and not in the ideas themselves.

It's hardly surprising that *Metamorphosis* became a wellspring from which much of radical, philosophical, psychiatry drank. Today, with reaffirmations of biological psychiatry we are inclined to see excessive intellectualisation as self-deceptive and a deviation from practical (helpful) interventions for psychotic people. At the same time, bringing existentialism into psychiatry broadened understanding of the experiences of schizophrenics, achieving a humanising response which was to try and understand *what it might be like*.

In this, radical practitioners were freed up by literature, enabled to avoid deciphering patients so as to better encounter them, their sensitivities and beliefs. With *Metamorphosis*, the link with psychosis is how it imputes states of isolation, of depersonalisation, of being unreal or of literally wasting or rotting away. At the centre of things crouches Gregor, his every corpuscle in a state of unconnectedness. However, this is no mere horror story and its symbolic repercussions sustain the overlay between the literary and what is. Says Anthony Thorlby (1972: 36): 'We have learned to recognise symbolism when we see it. And the symbolism of this story is plain: here is modern man in his alienated condition, treated as an insect by his fellows who think only of appearances.'

So too does psychosis carry inferences of outsider, provoking defensive isolation from those who seek conformity in behaviour and who employ seclusion, and where necessary, forced treatments to induce compliance. Yet we need to be wary about simple comparisons. Although they foster humanist perspectives: 'Literary masterpieces defy pat answers and do not yield to facile psychiatric interpreting or superficial diagnosing (Gans, 1998: 353).

In Kafka's narrative the inclination to jump from insect to schizophrenia is fed by its oddness, its improbability. Indeed, it is hard to avoid an element of authorial conceit in its entreaty to the reader to attach figurative meaning to its events. Perhaps that's what fiction is about, reformulating meanings in the service of other insights, different perspectives. Here is novelist William Trevor:

> The point is that the way a novel strikes critics and readers in general after I've written it is really up to them. They may find allegory … that I haven't put in and that wasn't my aim at all. But … it doesn't matter. That is what writing is all about. It's all about creating something which is then picked up by other people.
> (Del Rio Alvaro, 2006: 119)

Plausibility matters here however. To what extent can you pummel this or that meaning out a work of fiction? We know that Kafka's 'plots' elicit fanciful analysis but if the intellectual novel is about anything it is its resilience to different readings or, in the case of plays, diverse interpretation. That said, what of the core work itself? Is there anything about a play or novel that is definitive and/or resistant to different readings? What about a reading of *Metamorphosis*, transferred to the stage, where Gregor wakes up as Britney Spears? What price an audience's reaction to that? OK, fine, and one could merrily expand on this at length. The point though is that:

> It matters little to which [interpretation] one subscribes, as long as one does not loose sight of the story itself. The work of art, after all, is greater than the sum of its possible meanings, and this is deeply true of the *Metamorphosis*.
>   (Osborne, 1967: 40)

True, but contentious. I mean what about Marxist, Feminist, Postmodernist analyses which, say their advocates, amplify how literature is written, conceptualised and delivered? Harold Bloom (1998) calls these abridgers 'schools of resentment' hell-bent on destroying reading as a creative pleasure in its own right. To believe, sneers Bloom, that Marxist or Fascist interpretations of Shakespeare say anything interesting about Shakespeare – other than by accident – is a delusion, although such readings might reflect something about Marxism etc.

Nonetheless, literature *can* inform matters over and above preoccupations about literary theory or ideas. For instance, this book's premise is that fiction broadens understanding of mental illness, its origins and experience. Considering Gregor as psychotic, though, risks squeezing psychiatric significance from a story that's about much more. Still, as psychology students, it may still allow us to understand psychosis more insightfully, humanely and in its various social contexts.

The switch

Becoming a copy of oneself (to oneself) is bad enough. Changing into another species – be it wolf or insect – is simply annoying. In *Metamorphosis*, Kafka sensationally invokes this horror by turning Gregor, a travelling salesman, into a giant bug. The switch is quick, it's in the story's first sentence, it must be dealt with and it is (with dispiriting outcomes) deadpan style. We are asked to accept the transformation as not only possible but that it has happened and that the everyday nature of what follows – unreality measured by steady, declarative, prose – renders the stupendous believable. We all of us wake daily so as to awaken the world in turn. Here, the reverse occurs and what would otherwise be a bad dream – quickly shuddered off – assumes a reality to be faced and outfaced. So, poor Gregor. It's hard to know in God's name what he can do. I mean, any attempt to get out of this jam is going to make him look ridiculous. I mean, the *whole thing* is ridiculous. How can an insect (even a giant one) turn a key in a man-made lock? Such things can only end in disaster.

Why has Kafka convened this situation? I suppose to demonstrate how destructive conventional responses to 'unusualness' can be, although as well, and perhaps primarily, to show us how literature does or doesn't work. For the most part Gregor is the book's narrator. As such we see events from his vantage point, that of an insect hanging from a ceiling. It's a device that demonstrates the limits of fiction, for how better to suggest the awkwardness of 'the novelist' as observer than casting him as a narrator-insect. And the point is headed home by the matter-of-factness of a writing style that makes the unnatural appear normal. Although *Metamorphosis* is fantastical, possibly farcical, the practicalities of Gregor's situation dominate the action and it is this that drags us deeper into the story.

Pre-emptors

Others have considered the duality of human nature using quite different narrative methods. In Robert Louis Stevenson's *The Strange Case of Dr Jekyll and Mr Hyde* (1886/2002), for example, the changes implied are less about physical transformation and more the replacement of civility with malevolence but in a 'personage' still recognisably human. True, its gothic atmosphere cultivates an image of 'savage animal' but, actually, it was Rouben Mamoulian's (1931) film version that contrived this representation – as can happen with 'the film of the book'. Written during Queen Victoria's reign, Stevenson's novel mapped outward propriety against inward (suppressed) desire and the anxiolytic tensions that hold these in check. Victorian preoccupation with lust went hand in hand with concerns about madness – at the time construed as *split mind* – especially fears about 'the madman' as reptilian, at large, procreating insatiably. If Alex Comfort (1948: 9) is right that 'no form of art can be regarded in isolation from the society in which the artist lives' then be aware that *Jekyll and Hyde*, *Frankenstein*, and others of their ilk, came hot on the heels of Darwinian evolution where humans, descended from apes, carry their descent with them. So too did these novels follow upon Freudian claims of unconscious life, primeval forces that will wreak havoc if they break into consciousness. Freud had initially been influenced by Charcot and his experiments with hypnosis, experiments that also pointed towards duality in human nature.

Further, *Jekyll and Hyde* has us believe that when good and evil are proximal, then, ultimately, evil (the animalistic) wins out. That said, animals lack that consciousness which knows good from evil. The wolf attacks instinctively, not from vengeance or injustice, whereas Mr Hyde relishes depravity and its effects, even if this doesn't negate his human nature. Similarly, with the Steppenwolf (Harry Haller), redemptive elements are ever present, it's never an irreducible evil. Nevertheless, isn't it the absence of pathology that imbues inhumanity (in humans) with fascination? Doesn't the self-consciousness of evildoing render the doer perversely appealing, therein the magnetism of *Macbeth* (this volume, Chapter 9) and *Richard III* (this volume, Chapter 5)?

Discussing his work, novelist William Trevor (this volume, Chapter 8) states: 'Goodness is much less interesting to write about but it is a much more interesting quality in a person. Evil – a little bit in inverted commas – is much more fun' (Del Rio Alvaro, 2006: 122). By 'less interesting' Trevor means uncomplicated, that goodness defies overlay, that its effects are pretty obvious. Not for nothing do psychopaths jeer at the victims they silkily charm to their ruin.

The writer and his world

Like Hesse, Stevenson was influenced by Calvinist theology which preached that evil is *rooted* in the world, a belief embedded within European traditions in psychology, particularly psychoanalysis. Indeed, many of Stevenson's ideas originated in his dreams (see Jenni Calder's Introduction to the Penguin Classic's edition, 1999: 7–23, for an astute view on this.) These were the troubled origins of *Jekyll and Hyde*, its ambivalence towards evil and its doings. At the same time Stevenson presents evil as insidious, his novel building on sensations of dread that crawl through a city of shadows, crevices and alleyways: the city as metaphor, besieged by darkness. If Stevenson is right, that repressing desire is emotionally risky (a questionable assumption if one accepts the psychoanalytic claim that civilisation evolves from repression) then Harry Haller – Steppenwolf – is wise to trust both his instinct as well as his logic. But whatever the advantages of this duality Harry remains burdened with the misery it brings, as does Mr Hyde.

Many post-psychoanalytic critics adjudge dualistic concepts (or concepts of splitting) redundant, opting to see psychosis as a compound, jagged, fracture of the personality. In spite of this, comparisons with the dualism of Shakespeare, Hesse, Kafka and Stevenson can influence understandings of psychosis not just historically but contemporaneously as well. For example, the stigma and rejection that attach themselves to 'the madman', his assumed unpredictability, changeling nature, penchant for violence, *stem* from dualism. We see this in Macbeth, perplexed by how thoughts give rise to actions that follow but which he wishes didn't. Observing King Duncan's entrance into Macbeth's castle we watch civilisation turn to disorder, the 'sweet smelling air', as it breaches the castle, turning sour when inside, a place where 'nothing is but what is not', where atypical morality applies. In effect, Duncan has been admitted to a unit where duty unremittingly implodes into self-aggrandisement and vaulting ambition. Whether it be the internment of the mad in private attics or the mushrooming of asylums (private and public), a standard response to insanity has been to confine it and so adding to its gothic fascination. People like the boundaries that separate 'the mad' from 'civilisation' and imagination runs amok if boundaries are tampered with. Not for nothing did Elizabeth Shoenberg (1980) call mental hospitals 'castles of fantasy', their secretiveness a presentiment of the dangerousness within them. The cauldron as metamorphic: the stage as an empty space which accommodates compression, the human spirit 'cabined, cribbed, confined'. Macbeth's castle doesn't contain the violence but it does intensify its effects by seeming to. It's like seeing the world as an assembly line of images without beginning or end.

Psychiatricising *Metamorphosis*

According to Martin Amis, psychiatric explanations (of human affairs) are 'zero rudimentary'. So why does he concede their usefulness when judging his (sometimes fraught) relationship with his father? Needs must, I suppose. Try as we may, it becomes difficult not to psychiatricise life in general and a book like *Metamorphosis* cries out for it. For us, the temptation is to construe the story as an allegory for schizophrenia, a 'condition' whose Teflon capacity to defy interpretation is legendary. Indeed, for years different perceptions of mental distress have evolved in opposing ways and with important implications for patients.

But it was post-1960s radical psychiatry that exploded these differences controversially. In particular, the French philosopher/historian Michel Foucault popularised the idea that power was a locally controlled function – for example, he argued that medical language dominates treatment centres and that family power struggles inflict damage on their young. He also attacked capitalist systems stating that when individuals become useless to them they are shunted aside as 'unknown aliens' (the original name for psychiatrist was *alienist*) and reassigned an identity of 'madness'. Forced to sustain an identity within the straightjacket of institutionalisation – whether by lock and key and/or diagnosis – the individual acts to diminish the demands made upon him, and where even success will entail massive concessions to conformity. Pfeiffer (1962: 57) aligns this with Gregor's position.

> The metamorphosed Gregor Samsa, having dropped out of the system of coordinates of normal existence, having been irrevocably removed from everything that constitutes life, exhausts himself in constantly renewed efforts to retain a connection with this existence until he gradually resigns himself and finally perishes.

Post-1960s radical psychiatrists positioned the psychotic at the margins of family life. They believed that the genesis of psychosis was existential horror consequent on an individual's realisation of cognitive disjunction with a threatening surroundings. This led ultimately (and unsustainably) to a standpoint whereby the schizophrenic was perceived as a primitive philosopher embarking on a voyage of self-fulfilment. R.D. Laing opened Kingsley Hull in London, a community where psychotic people met with psychiatrists (literally around a banquet table) and philosophised, no doubt aided and abetted by diverse stimuli, into the night. The disposition to enquire into the meaning of things had the moral effect of rendering 'the schizophrenic' less passive, actually worthy of enquiry and interest. This was fine as it went. However, its problematic contention that psychosis was not just perpetuated but induced by family life caused offence to the families of mentally ill people.

However, the biggest mistake of anti-psychiatry was to affirm 'the family' as an abstract entity without recourse to actual families in terms of class, culture, economics and so forth. With very little evidence 'the family' was damned as a pernicious system of graduated dehumanisation and emasculation. The mechanism ran something like this: within the matrix of a family, one of its young succumbs to parent driven guilt-inducing accusations, constant reminders of unworthiness and ineffectuality. Based on observations of eleven families, psychiatrists R.D. Laing and Aaron Esterson, (Laing & Esterson, 1964: 7) outlined their theory of schism:

> If one wishes to know how a football team concert or disconcert their actions in a play, one does not think only, or even primarily, of approaching this problem by talking to the members individually, one watches the way they play together. Most of the investigations of families of schizophrenics, whilst contributing original useful data to different facets of the problem, have not been based on direct observation of the members of the family *together* as they actually interact with each other.

Unusual for its time, the sources of this thinking were taken from continental philosophy, mainly Foucault, Heidegger, but also Kafka, as Laing (1960: 41) would point out:

> Shakespeare's world, quite as much as Kafka's, is that prison cell which Pascal says the world is, from which daily the inmates are led forth to die; [this] forces upon us the cruel irrationality of the conditions of human life, the tale told by an idiot.

But in Kafka, before Gregor dies, something is done to him. This victimisation of individuals (before death) is standard Kafka, and the victim's friends, if she/ he has any, are usually of the fair-weather kind, a factor that helps us understand schizophrenia, if not its causation then at least as a lived experience.

In retrospect, the radical psychiatrists confused cause-and-effect with correlation. That is, observing the debilitating effects of parenting on the young they instanced this as causal when actually it was exacerbation. In other words, and as we now know from Julian Leff's studies (Leff & Vaughn, 1980), negative criticism does induce deterioration in psychotic people, but the psychotic state may already be present. Although *Metamorphosis* was read by radical psychiatrists, they too readily seized on its resemblances to their theories on families, ignoring what was contradictory.

Actually, defining Gregor's state as a family-induced psychosis poses several problems. Pfeiffer (1962: 56), for instance, challenges any analysis that begins with the Samsa family. pointing out that we see events courtesy of Gregor and that 'any attempt to disregard this, so vital for the meaning of the whole story, to transfer the centre of gravity to the family amounts to arbitrary distortion'. Moreover, *Metamorphosis* illustrates a family *just like any other,* a reasonably structured unit, economically interdependent and psychosociologically average. To begin with, Gregor's family is loving and his father, traditionally the breadwinner, has kept the family viable, contented, well knit. But when the son assumes economic responsibility, the father turns resentful and, unable to cope with this reaction as well as his new responsibilities, Gregor collapses. In this respect Kafka shows how the vicissitudes of family life incur meanings, perceptions, and irregularities inclusive of a particular family's notions of what family life should be. Shades of Tolstoy's dictum: 'Happy families are all alike: every unhappy family is unhappy in its own way'.

The family

Kafka knew that families inflicted psychological damage on one or other of their members. His novel watches the Samsas closely and especially how their beliefs, values and emotions change in line with Gregor becoming a bug. Until then Gregor has been the 'white-haired boy' providing for his family dutifully, necessarily so given the loss of his father's business and the family's mounting debts. Nothing remarkable about that: until *it* happens, until the change occurs whereby nothing is ever the same again. We discover Gregor's 'good boy' status retrospectively but from it we can see his transformation as liberating, an escape from the drudgery of ensuring the family's (financial) stability. At the same time, his transformation limits their dependence such that they are now free to behave towards him as they wish.

For us, it is precisely the absurdity of his position that allows entry to its unthinkable implications. From his place in the narrative we access events from *inside his room.* For example, we are preoccupied by Gregor's itemised notation of the things that surround him such that when an outside narrator intrudes it's almost a relief. When Gregor enters the *family* room, however, panic ensues and an 'outside' narrator informs us of his filthy state and for a moment we see Gregor as others do. And when at the end he dies, it is the extra narrator who makes the story cohere, the novel's premise made effective.

The locked door

Anyone that worked in the hospitals/asylums will recall locked doors and the significance (metaphorical and real) of 'holding the keys'. Having, from the 1950s, enjoyed a lengthy period of open doors within our mental health system (Clarke, 2004) locks and locking are back with a vengeance. With the advent of forensic units, particularly, there now prevails, as at the turn of the last century, an excessive concern about aggression and its containment.

What does being 'locked in' entail? Is the locked door a safety barrier by which patients test their psychological and interpersonal resilience, a buffer against the effects of their actions on others? Or does it, as Goffman (1968) suggests, constitute a totalising boundary that induces obedience, conformity, as well as the imagined dangers of what lies beyond the doors: better to be locked in and safe than free but sorry?

Why is Gregor's bedroom door locked? What purpose is served in its being locked? Is it by force of habit? What can he fear from his family? Does he see them as potential aggressors? In Joseph Heller's *Something Happened* (1974: 3), Bob Slocum confesses:

> I get the willies when I see closed doors. Even at work, where I am doing so well now, the sight of a closed door is sometimes enough to make me dread that something horrible is happening behind it, something that is going to affect me adversely; if I am tired and dejected ... I can almost smell the disaster mounting invisibly and flooding out toward me through the frosted glass panes. My hands may perspire, and my voice may come out strange. I wonder why. Something must have happened to me sometime.

This is the anxiety endemic to corporate life: the 'rat race', the pressure to *perform*, to do something well that is itself unwell, the dread that something has or *is* happening of which one knows little or nothing but which is going down all the same. In his review of *Something Happened,* 'this astonishingly pessimistic novel', Kurt Vonnegut (1974: 11) surmised that: 'Depictions of utter hopelessness in literature have been acceptable up to now only in small doses, in short-story form, as in Franz Kafka's *Metamorphosis.*'

Like Gregor, we don't know what Bob Slocum is guilty of: he's guilty of something, that's for sure, but what? They're corporate men and they appear to take on too much responsibility for things. Innocence is lost and that which takes its place is not nice in any sense: the family especially, that ought to be in harmony, mutually respectful, loving, is so for a time but then things fall apart and a kind of hatred or unknowingness of each other arises.

Perhaps the difference is that in *Metamorphosis* the anxiety is about what has yet to be attained. We know that clinical anxiety takes two forms. Firstly, 'free floating', with people unable to rationalise their sense of an impending doom. Something – what? – lurks beyond the twist of time such that they are forever crossing the bridges of life far in advance of reaching them. Secondly, anxiety is phobic, fear of everyday objects but which objects are metaphors for: what? When Gregor locks his door, what does he fear lies behind it? Mesmerised, we watch him try to turn the key in the lock, the hilariousness of which Muir observes (1964: 39):

> evokes the imperfection of all human arrangements … the humour here is the kind that rises from the contemplation of pedantically conscientious inefficiency; every action is perfectly reasonable yet, except to the actors, senselessly absurd. It is really a hackneyed music-hall type of turn, the sort we laugh at when we see a comedian frenziedly trying to do two jobs at the same time.

This is the laughter that attends absurdity censuring what is not straightforwardly comprehensible. Gregor's efforts at turning the key reflect the desperation of breaching the boundary of his room. The incongruity heightens the conflicts intrinsic to the spaces between self and physical containment. Maybe the inmates of forensic units should read *Metamorphosis*. It might dislodge the psychological justification – containment is safe and therefore liberating – that sustains incarceration. This novel is key to exploring the experience of detention and its ramifications for all concerned. What does restricted space mean for staff as well as patients and how is space used given how time passes within it? Living through time as an inmate is akin to watching the proverbial kettle boil whilst inside it. Time slows, life becomes interminable and with aggression a relief-giving valve from monotony, the violent act discharging all reason between aggressor and adversary, the intensity splitting apart the core of the enclosed space.

In *Macbeth*, madness is evil and evil is the cosmos. Cataclysmic forces – compressed within a castle, arranged on a stage – impel actions that have awful consequences. Gregor's room is the cosmos, an implosive gap between which struggles Everyman and unhappiness, but, like Bob Slocum, why should he be unhappy, why has 'something happened'? Perhaps in the Samsa household time and space have collapsed so that what transpires is universally significant: enclosed spaces – like forensic cells – have the effect of warping time and memory, confusing wakefulness and dreams. In *Macbeth,* distance is traversed psychologically as when Lady Macbeth broadcasts her thoughts to her husband. So, from inside Gregor's room, does the terribleness of his dissidence invoke those competing forces of corporate and personal power that constitute our lives.

Daddy dearest

In Kafka's stories, as in his life, there is always a father figure to be assuaged. Indeed, this was an artist who had 'gone on past boyhood accepting the role of cockroach for which, like the hero of *Metamorphosis,* he had been cast by the bourgeois' (Wilson, 1962: 94) of which Papa was exemplary. Convinced he had not measured up to his father's expectations he berated himself for this. When he was dying he asked Max Brod to destroy his work and we may surmise this as the unconscious wish for the death of the father which is to say that those (Hawes, 2008) challenging the genuineness of Kafka's request are somewhat missing the point. The relationship of father and son had been tense and unresolved, and this spills into the novel. Four years after completing *Metamorphosis* – and still living with his parents – Kafka (1919) wrote a 100-page letter to his father. In it, Kafka proclaims a fear of his father but which, he says, is unfathomable and difficult to articulate. He confesses to never having interested himself in his father's affairs preferring the secrecy and safety of his room. It's not that he is unaware of his father's shortcomings but that his father's temperament so contradicts his own. Paternal disapproval eventually led to his entertaining 'feelings of being nothing'. On a swimming expedition he recalled, 'There was I, skinny, weakly, slight; you strong, tall, broad … I felt a miserable specimen not only in your eyes but in the eyes of the whole world, for you were for me the measure of all things.'

Later, he relates how, on the receiving end of paternal rage – 'I will tear you apart like a fish!' – he lost the capacity to talk, a motif that underwrites the novel, that survival depends heavily on the capacity for 'normal' conversation. On and on the letter goes, its agonised construction fully apparent, at times berating his father whilst incessantly self-recriminating and seemingly incapable of controlling his own life. At one point he declares that he is a bachelor because he *cannot* marry: that is, 'I'm not the marrying kind'. Why? Because the qualities that sustain marriage are (surprise, surprise) those possessed by his father 'warts and all'. So Gregor has worked his tail end off though we discover that money has been in the family all along, money held over from the past. Also, isn't it strange that the family employs servants – and exactly why can't the father work anymore?

Much of the letter sounds familiar. Terrible paternal condemnations of the 'when I was your age I had to do this or that' kind or 'you young people don't know you're born today' and so on. Franz's response is passive at first but he quickly learns to poke fun at his father's pomposity and grandstanding. It was this, he says, that allowed him not only to escape paternal derision but to free himself up from his family altogether. For whatever the kindnesses he had enjoyed from his mother or sister, these too came indirectly through Daddy's patronage, a not uncommon arrangement at the time. This is the family background from which *Metamorphosis* sprung and whilst the novel is hardly autobiographical it does carry Kafka's anxieties of being treated disparagingly because different, because of failing to live up to standards. In this, his work illuminates the apprehension of what it might be like to undergo profound change whilst remaining sentient of the difference.

A dream

Psychiatrist Jerome Gans (1998) believes that therapists will gain insights and competencies from reading *Metamorphosis* and similar texts. He argues that assigning feelings to others can characterise the existence of others as if it were one's own. Such a process, however, involves a massive depletion resulting in an inability to accept future events as one's own responsibility. With Gregor, it is his father who is to blame for his inability to marry: 'for I would have to be like my father to do so'. But perhaps he is unlike his father because he has *made* his father into something he isn't. So may his helplessness fuel aggression, an emotion that rarely works better than when expressed: 'help me, please, please help *me*' and one has seen patients inflict this on therapists with barely hidden glee. As Gans (p. 362) notes, an empathic stance towards Gregor or indeed this schismatic family is not always easy and the story as it proceeds becomes an excellent lesson in the fragility of empathic responding. For many of us, our responses to Gregor and the others will waver and change but how true is this too of working with clients, and at least the novel is fodder for reflection on the difficulties and intransigencies involved.

Such ideas cannot be tested of course and inasmuch as we take different experiences from books so as therapists do we 'read' patients differently. Because pretensions of expertise or brash self-assurance are *the* endemic temptation for neophyte therapists, reading *Metamorphosis* becomes a master class in appraising ambiguity. Its perplexity challenges students to examine their reactions to what at first glance is a morbid fairy tale but which is really a story steeped in irony, obfuscation, bad turnings and dead ends.

Contemporary psychiatry champions biology, pharmacology and a second-hand therapy (cognitive behaviourism) derived from learning theory. In such a climate it's good to re-enervate notions of mental distress as complex, elusive and deserving of philosophical enquiry. Equally, it becomes important to emphasise the relevance of patient's narratives to recovery: even to *partly* disregard this aspect of care is unforgivable. Taking account of literature precludes easy assumptions about behaviour, assumptions that mandate responses – 'techniques' – that exhibit the hallmarks of superficiality, received ideas, and an alignment with economics and generating 'patient output'. Of course most of us would prefer patient outcomes better than those which befall Gregor: how nice it would have been had he lost his worries and made his way in the world, even at the expense – within limits – of others. However, *Metamorphosis* 'makes the reader experience the events as if they were present, especially in the sense that they have the incoherence of the present and do not point to an outcome' (Pascal, 1982: 39).

It is a wise psychiatry that recognises that there are no outcomes necessarily more pleasant than the present state of things and that this is worth understanding whether in therapy or otherwise. The discernment that *Metamorphosis* provides is about the inexplicability of much human reaction and the disappointment that comes from not having clear – resolved – outcomes. It's a novel that creates its own realm demonstrating the limitless expansion of humanness and its defiance of simplistic comprehension. In our psychological work this behoves us to look beyond the prism of scientific investigation for it's surely fatuous to suppose we need scientific training to *appreciate* our surroundings. Biochemistry has its place but there is a higher order understanding that encompasses both behaviour *and* biochemistry in any of their relationships.

That we exist in the world in different ways demands tolerance. Psychosis is a severe test of tolerance, it affects all who come near it, especially families. *Metamorphosis* is testimony to how adverse, judgemental, conditions, expressed by families or wider social groups, may be experienced and faced up to. Psychiatrists Phil Thomas and Pat Bracken (1999: 11) state that 'by definition, psychosis involves a person being in a state whereby ordinary, accepted, reality is put into question. The experience of time, space and the coherence of the world becomes fragile.'

We wonder at Gregor's lost capacity to act on things as he used to. Those around him have tried to help him but in piecemeal fashion, attempting to work around him, changing his immediate environment and so on. But nothing has worked. The one thing missing is the effort to engage with *him*, with the terror of the nature of his alteration. It is lack of regard that kills him but it's hardly anyone's fault if one is being asked to care for something no longer human, something grotesque. Is it?

Films

Metamorphosis was televised in 1987 by actor/director Steven Berkoff and produced by the BBC. It was based on Berkoff's stage production first performed at the Roundhouse in 1969. A copy of his 'script' (Berkoff, 2000) – most of the action was mimed – is available. Berkoff's conception of Gregor is that he is always a little outside of his family, always watching and waiting. 'This frightened human being', he has said, 'touched me in all my chords of being from grotesque to simple.' The production still plays to audiences all over the world.

In 2006 a British theatre director, David Farr, and an Icelandic actor/director Gisli Orn Gardarrson began working on a stage version. The production stunned European audiences with its literal portrayal of Gregor and his predicament. Gardarrson, also a circus acrobat, performs a series of amazing movements across and along scaffolding as he tries to cope with his altered physical state. The script stays very close to the novel and Gardarrson's hoarseness personifies stricken Gregor's 'failure to communicate' memorably. The music score, by rock artist Nick Cave (with Warren Ellis), is innovative and startling. The production company is called Vesturport and we can only wait eagerly for a film version.

References

Bateson, G, Jackson DD, Haley, J & Weakland J (1956) Towards a theory of schizophrenia. *Behavioural Science,1*, 251–64.

Berkoff, S (2000) *Three Plays*. London: Faber & Faber.

Bloom, H (1998) *The Invention of the Human*. New York: Riverhead Books.

Calder, J (1999) *The Strange Case of Dr Jekyll and Mr Hyde*. London: Penguin Classics.

Clarke, L (2004) *The Time of the Therapeutic Communities*. London: Jessica Kingsley.

Comfort, A (1948) *The Novel and Our Time*. London: Phoenix House.

Cooper, D (1972) *The Death of the Family*. Harmondsworth: Penguin.

Del Rio Alvaro, C (2006) Talking with William Trevor: It all seems natural now. *Estudio Irlandeses, 1*, 119–24.

Gans, JS (1998) Narrative lessons for the psychotherapist: Kafka's 'The Metamorphosis'. *American Journal of Psychotherapy, 52* (3), 352–66.

Goffman, E (1960) *Asylums*. Harmondsworth: Penguin.

Hawes, J (2008) *Excavating Kafka*. London: Quercus.

Heller, J (1974) *Something Happened*. London: Jonathan Cape.

Kafka, F (1919) *Letter to His Father*. Available online at: http://www.kafka-franz.com/KAFKA-letter.htm

Kafka, F (1999) *Metamorphoses and Other Stories*. London: Vintage.

Kott, J (1967) *Shakespeare: Our contemporary*. London: Methuen.

Kuna, F (1974) *Kafka: Literature as corrective punishment*. London: Paul Elek.

Laing, RD (1960) *The Divided Self*. London: Tavistock.

Laing, RD & Esterson, A (1964) *Sanity, Madness and the Family*. London: Tavistock.

Leff, J & Vaughn, CE (1980) The interaction of life events and relatives' expressed emotions in schizophrenia and depressed neurosis. *British Journal of Psychiatry, 136*, 146–53.

Mamoulian, R (1931) *Dr Jekyll and Mr Hyde* [film]. Hollywood: Warner Home Movies.

Muir, E (1964) Franz Kafka. In R Gray (ed), *A Collection of Critical Essays* (pp 33–44). Englewood Cliffs, NJ: Prentice-Hall.

Nabokov, V (1980) *Lectures on Literature*. London: Harcourt.

Nagel, T (1974) What is it like to be a bat? *The Philosophical Review, 83*(4), 435–50.

Osborne, C (1967) *Kafka*. Edinburgh: Oliver & Boyd.

Pascal, R (1982) *Kafka's Narrators*. Cambridge: Cambridge University Press.

Pasley, M (1963) *Short Stories*. Oxford: Oxford University Press.

Pfeiffer, J (1962) The metamorphosis. In R Gray (ed), *Kafka: A collection of critical essays* (pp 33–9). Englewood Cliffs, NJ: Prentice Hall.

Shoenberg, E (1980) Therapeutic communities: The ideal, the real and the possible. In E Jansen (ed) *The Therapeutic Community* (pp 64–71). Englewood Cliffs, NJ: Croom Helm.

Stevenson, RL (2002) *The Strange Case of Dr Jekyll and Mr Hyde*. Harmondsworth: Penguin. [Original work published 1886]

Thomas, P & Bracken, P (1999) Science, psychiatry and the mystery of madness. *Openmind, 100,* 10–11.

Thorlby, A (1972) *A Student's Guide to Kafka*. London: Heinemann Educational.

von Sacher-Masoch, L (2006) *Venus in Furs*. Harmondsworth: Penguin Classics. [Original work published 1870]

Vonnegut, K (1974) 'Something Happened' Review. *New York Times Book Review, 11,* 6 October.

Wilson, E (1962) A dissenting opinion on Kafka. In R Gray (ed), *Kafka: A collection of critical essays* (pp 91–7). Englewood Cliffs, NJ: Prentice-Hall.

FELICIA'S JOURNEY

Think your escaping and run into yourself.
Longest way round is the shortest way home.
  (James Joyce, *Ulysses*)

For Atom Egoyan's (1999) film version of William Trevor's *Felicia's Journey* the publicity blurb reads 'monsters aren't born'. Whether this is to expiate Mr. Hildich, the monster in the story, or a testament to social determinants of human evil, is an open question and best addressed from within the novel. After all, that is the point (of this book), that literature yields certain insights closed down by formal medical tracts. This is especially true of what has been traditionally diagnosed as 'psychopathy', 'sociopathy' or 'personality disorder', the diagnosis that psychiatry is most uncomfortable with, essentially because it lacks psychotic symptoms but, as well, is beset by problems that are asocial, moral, criminal. In the main, it is the issue of morality that is conceptually most difficult because it flags up the role of evil in human intention. Psychiatry, posing as an objective science, can hardly talk about good and evil but fiction does this in spades. In Trevor's work, evil comes about through vulnerability, naïveté and chance but, as we shall see, is ultimately overcome or at least tempered by civility and forgiveness.

Set in the 1990s, *Felicia's Journey* is told against clashing cultures. It's a kind of 'innocents abroad' saga with England a land studded with soulless factory estates, its streets littered with the debris of vulgar affluence, not a very nice place to be. Enter Felicia, an Irish girl, lost, gullible, impregnated by a 'Paddy' who has joined the British army. A product of an Irish Catholic nationalist family she has come to England to find him, only he has lied to her about his whereabouts and his occupation. She encounters a Mr Hilditch who seemingly wants to take her under his wing and who, we soon discover, has already taken other girls into his care, of whom nothing more is known, apart from how he remembers them within the story. Thus do matters proceed, embodied within the two main characters, as a story of Irish innocence stained by English malevolence. In these terms some have seen *Felicia's Journey* as a 'write-back', postcolonial, novel whose sub-text is the settling of political/historical scores. But it's not only this. Trevor knows the complexities of Irish-British history, particularly that ageless Irish talent to incessantly 'blame the others'. So that *Felicia's Journey* is less a postcolonial novel, more now-colonial, its basic theme of innocence corrupted by cynicism set within a modern framework.

That said, Trevor's description of Ireland can seem winsomely outdated, his use of male stage-Irish names: 'Dirty Keery', 'Artie Slattery', 'Old Begley', 'Tim Bo Gargin', 'Small Crowley', sounding quaint in contemporary terms. Yet despite these clichéd 'ould Ireland' labels, *Felicia's Journey* presents uncomfortable truths at odds with (in some Irish quarters) a pretentious modernism that seeks to camouflage a perceived primitivism of the past by assertions of bogus sophistication. Luke Gibbons (1996: 83) however provides an accurate picture of the Ireland from which Felicia starts her journey:

> The chronic unemployment ... the demoralisation in the aftermath of the abortion and divorce referenda, the growth of a new underclass, the re-appearance of full scale emigration, the new censorship mentality and, not least, the moving statues, constituted a return of the repressed for those intent on bringing Ireland into the modern world. If a Rip Van Winkle fell asleep in the 1950s and woke up in 1988, he could be forgiven for thinking that nothing had changed in between.

So that although Trevor, himself an emigrant (to England), brought with him a distinctive (if criticised) 1950s vision of Ireland, this actually carried a good deal of sustainable truth. The fact is, values change laboriously, unlike fashions and outward appearance, such that Trevor's Ireland is:

> a bleak place where people endure life rather than live it; a place of loneliness, frustration and undramatic suffering. Timeless, except in its details, its moral climate remains constant whether its people live in the 1940s or the 1990s.
> (MacKenna, 1999: 139)

So in transporting his 'heroine' to an English milieu, there crystallises interpersonal tensions, difficult to articulate, because Hilditch and Felicia hold very different ambitions. He is deceptive and manipulative whereas she, immunised by an 'old Ireland' mentality against worldliness and relativism, is increasingly befuddled. But so what? Is there a problem with unworldliness or in rejecting relativism for absolutism whether political or moral in kind? In his Nobel Prize-winning speech, Seamus Heaney (1995) began by saying that as a small boy in late 1940s Derry he never dreamed that he would ever see a city like Stockholm, much less be welcomed to it as a Nobel Laureate. As a child in a large family, he recalls how they:

> crowded together in three rooms of a traditional thatched farmstead and lived a kind of den life which was more or less intellectually proofed against the outside world. It was an intimate, physical, creaturely, existence in which the night sounds of the horse in the stable beyond one bedroom wall mingled with the sounds of adult conversation from the kitchen beyond the other ... ahistorical, pre-sexual, in suspension between the archaic and the modern.

Yet as time passed so did Heaney's faculties sharpen; the 'small things' of life forging a poetry that would deservedly win universal approbation. But not all possess the poetic muse and in Felicia we meet someone in whom the mores of an inward-looking family and community, which at one level she has rejected, persevere in her consciousness. For Felicia, there will be no flight into poetics or other intellectual salvation although ultimately serenity will come from the kinship of street persons, a blessed vagrancy.

Two tribes

In fact, Trevor's upbringing comprised both traditions of Irish history, the Protestant landed gentry of his middle-class family but, as well, an awareness of poor rural Irishness. This mixed lineage is what gives him an outsider capacity to see the myriad variables of both traditions. In addition, he considers his residence in Devon these past fifty or so years an observational bonus.

> Trevor approaches his creations with detachment, with an ironic distance nevertheless always balanced by compassion so that the reader can always feel the fragility and humanity of even the most evil of his characters.
> (Del Rio Alvaro, 2007: 2)

That is, Trevor is a moralist whose work encircles evil, madness and alienation. This is not to say that he moralises, far from it; but what he does do is illustrate how ordinariness attends violent, murderous, acts, how, in the minutiae of simply 'getting through' the day, there lurk horrendous dangers. Embedded in the detail of people wanting to connect but not being able to, or at least not in ways that are loving or even pleasurable, abides the genesis of destruction. 'Still waters run deep' is but one of a hundred euphemisms that describes the inexplicable conjunction of the quiet neighbour, 'who wouldn't hurt a fly' but who hurts far more, and then some. The shock of evil 'that lies beneath' is how it disturbs the comforts found in more extreme imagery; the more gruesome, the more strangely comforting (because surreally unreal). So have 'psychopaths' been paraded in literature and cinema as fantastical, for example, the gurning antics of Jack Torrance in Kubrick's *The Shining* (1980) or the 'over the top' flashiness of Hannibal Lecter in Harris's (1988) *Silence of the Lambs*. As Cynthia Fuchs (2008) notes: 'Serial killers ... are best known for their sensational styles: they wear knife-fingered gloves, hockey masks, or cheesy Halloween costumes', they film or tape their crimes or, in *The Butcher Boy* (McCabe, 1992), commemorate slaughter with the blood smeared like an insignia, across the walls of their victims. These are the sorts you don't want to meet on a dark night. But at least if you did, you'd have some inkling of impending trouble. Not so with Joseph Ambrose Hilditch, the beneficent uncle, the 'good Samaritan', the rotund 'daddy', the dispenser of benign assurance.

Telling the story

Trevor is a master of authorial unobtrusiveness. Not for him the trickery of postmodernist flitting within, around and outside narrative. Instead, his is the time-honoured tradition of novel writing, realism. Dickens is an influence as is Jane Austen, Anthony Powell and Graham Greene. So would Kingsley Amis have been proud of Trevor's style if not quite at ease with his content. However, praising Trevor's attention to detail risks undervaluing his agility at psychological analysis. Deftness in fiction writing is now unfashionable and in much Irish writing of late there has broken out a flamboyance of form and content for which Trevor has little time (in this respect, see the novels of Roddy Doyle, 1987, 1991 or Neil Jordan, 1983, 2005). Trevor instead deals with a world we know but, by slipping in the unexpected, he shows how things can go awry and seriously so at that. 'God moves in mysterious ways' as Miss Calligary would say, and it's worth pondering what might have happened had she not stumbled upon Felicia and Mr Hilditch. Nothing is forced here, it's simply the case that stuff happens. States Anne Duchene, Trevor: 'takes the known world, makes his comment, and leaves the mixture just slightly sourer than before' (cited in Duguid, 2002: 296). In terms of character it's a technique that builds in elements that are at once evil incarnate but with room left over for pity and recovery.

Hilditch

Hilditch is a most conventional man. A catering manager respected by employers and underlings alike, he lives in a residential area named after one of Britain's greatest generals. Perhaps it's a bit odd that he has never married but there again he doesn't seem bothered. He shaves closely, dresses as a middle-class man would and he appears to like being liked. Which is all a bit dull (not that he'd mind that either) as well as self-contained, not connected up, humourless, hidden.

Mr. Hilditch is fastidious. Concerned not to 'dirty his own doorstep', he has a rule never to be seen near his place of work or his neighbourhood with the young ladies he befriends. 'People talk' and he doesn't want anyone getting the wrong idea. He's a skilful conversationalist, a questioner, constantly probing, flattering, working out 'the lay of the land'. Observe how he repeats Felicia's name when talking to her, as well, his manipulative use of silence. He is, as well, *a skilful smiler*. From the start, we are suspicious of what or who he is, for when alone, Trevor (1995: 7) tells us, he: 'is often brought closer to other, darker, aspects of the depths that lie within him. When a smile no longer matters he can be a melancholy man.'

Obsessional, he needs things in their place including people whom he either invents or collects and, in his case, there is the invention of a military past so as to feed his supremacist view of England's history. The preoccupation with pasts includes hanging old photos and portraits of strangers on his walls. He is a rejected Mummy's boy unable to let (his late) Mummy go. His memories of her general promiscuousness disturbs him as does the sexual abuse – Trevor isn't explicit here – which represses his rage at not possessing Mummy the way that Uncle Wilf did.

Freudian psychology asserts that if we know 'the child' we can calculate the man. From a clinical perspective this means that childhood trauma may claw its way to psychological abnormality in adulthood. This, although pessimistic, fails to address adequately a concept of evil, or its effects. For that, we best turn to Freud's disciple Carl Jung and his 'collective unconscious', which invokes a mythology of original sin, the seminal 'fall' in the Garden of Eden and the resulting propensity to do evil. And, consistent with original sin, Trevor focuses on characters who are themselves players in their own distress. At different points Felicia tells us that she knows her journey is fruitless so that, in real terms, her crossing the Irish Sea is less about the 'facts of the case' and more a drifting towards self-knowledge and fulfilment.

Pursuant of Catholic theology where we all of us bear the stain of original sin, there can be redemption for those who ask, and do penance, for it. But this is a process of becoming in which inevitably something – perhaps sometimes remembered and cherished – is lost. In this book, characters navigate life under pressure, communicating to us, less so to one another, life's significant events as they encounter them. Hilditch engineers situations, far from home base where, an unlikely Don Juan, he can be appraised as the putative lover of whichever girl he happens to be with, that people will see these girls as his sexual conquests arouses him. And yet he never mentions having had sex with them (or killing them). Having repressed his aggressive sexuality he rationalises events such that killing the girls is warped into what he calls 'the ending of a friendship'. By killing them, he gives them innocence, saves them from sin and degradation, filth, the bogs: repressing this affords him a measure of civility, of self-regard. What's wrong in being cruel to be kind and, besides, they asked for it, didn't they? Innocence excites people like Hilditch, the psychopath's gratification is at its utmost when predatory, when taking from others what is rightfully theirs, whether intellectually, emotionally or literally.

Felicia

'I don't know, am I in the right place?' (p. 11) says Felicia, Irish vernacular for 'I don't know if I am in the right place', one of a million or more Irish voices that stumbled from the ferries at Holyhead port. Hilditch knowingly fingers her as someone at sixes and sevens but more so as Irish, a condition that repels him. Her presence kick-starts his memories of British superiority, days of Empire, military might and army uncles sent to Ireland to 'read the riot act' and sort 'the paddies' out. To Hilditch, Ireland is 'a bogland' and this plays to his secret desires insofar as preventing Felicia from going back will save her from: 'A fate which is, literally worse than death and one from which he, the enlightened colonial redeemer, must deliver her, the misguided postcolonial victim'(St Peter, 2002: 336).

But he knows that she's different from the others, that there's nothing tough about her: 'simple as a bird, which you'd expect her to be of course, coming from where she does. And yet, of course, they're all the same. The truth stares out at them and they avert their eyes' (p. 127). This is a passage of contradiction and denial. Mr Hilditch, a man of imperial tastes, equates Felicia's simplicity with Ireland, the land of 'the bogs' and where people are intellectually diminished. And yet, he says, she's no different from his other girls and their 'street-wise' ways, they all know the score. Yet were this true, had Felicia been more assured about men, less naïve about the discomfort of strangers, had she not come from a relatively closed community, things might have turned out differently. Yet, having said that, the other girls *did* have the urban knowledge Felicia lacked, were more worldly wise, sexually aware. So something more than a normative concept of interpersonal relationships and psychology seems needed to account for what befalls them.

Our current psychiatric culture craves explanations for whatever phenomena we confront and we are uncomfortable with that which resists explanation. As psychologists we endless construct models in the effort to 'frame' behaviour in the expectation that in naming things we can believe their existence and therefore control them. So, in our current climate, do we seek to build up evidence-based practices – in the sense of material-quantitative evidence – partly as a factor of accountability but, also, as a resistance to what might generally be called 'the intractable'. Things happen that are difficult to account for possibly because only dimly apprehended and some people put themselves in harm's way for other, equally indiscernible, reasons.

Nationalism

Living as an immigrant in a host culture that claims ascendancy over one's native traditions is problematic. Felicia carries within her the arch symbol of that ascendancy, a child of the British military. Inside her republican background, this is something that usually merits revulsion and she has indeed been so reviled by her aggrieved father.

However, a degree of ambivalence attends this nationalism. The old woman of 100 years represents Gaelic history, fittingly so for a land that often mythologizes itself as 'Mother Ireland'. Felicia's father, who concretises this history in newspaper cut-outs and speeches, has the job of narrating Ireland's past against 'the British' whose responsibility for Irish failures are, as he sees it, conspicuous and dastardly. Her father's speech (p. 58) has a flavour of the postcolonial novel, capturing well the explosive political interjections of that genre. However, on reading this speech one is struck by its impulsiveness, its sense of neither having been thought through very much or deeply felt. Its sense is of a list of slogans dredged from a past that has lost much of its significance to a good many, especially young, people. Thus does Trevor encase a bunch of contrived epithets within an irony that shows their political redundancy, in effect, a jingoism widely missing the mark of Felicia's problems and whose solutions lie in the personal. Political, social and historical baggage is not irrelevant but is subsidiary to those who must carry it but who didn't choose it.

The perversity of language

Felicia's Journey is packed with contradictions, incongruities and enigmas. Felicia's errant lover is Irish but wears a British army uniform, is disreputable and an accomplished liar. Mr Hilditch is an even bigger liar, a fantasist soldier of imperialist proportions. Yet he seems less annoyed by Johnny Lysaght's British army jacket than by the innocent 'boglander' who he thinks deserves what she gets. The Irishness is repugnant, but its embodiment as female gullibility is what really irks him. Trevor seems to idealise women, for all of the men here are insensitive and given over to violence. Though he repents, Felicia's father calls her a whore and her brothers are allowed no more fictional space than to display their capacity for violence in the settling of a score.

No one in the book tells the truth either and nobody listens if someone tries to. Felicia and Hilditch talk over one another, each preoccupied with different things. An example of this talking over and/or against is the dialogue between Miss Calligary and the old lady (pp. 78–81). Whilst appearing to carry on the rudiments of discussion they are utterly at odds with each other to a degree that is almost surreal. It's a technique of overlapping dialogue that Trevor uses a lot and none more subtly than when Hilditch and Felicia talk at each other. Caught up in their own reveries, carrying their imaginations of pasts and future possibilities on their backs, the effect is of nobody listening to anyone.

Here are people so fatally linked that interchanges between them are simply a going through the motions as though inside a dream. It's as though something has brought them together in the service of some purpose that is being worked towards but which is difficult to identify. And actually, that is the sense one gets reading this book. That is, until near the end. Entering Felicia's bedroom (pp. 153–6) when she *is* in a dream Hilditch shatters it with disclosures which now allow her to see him for what he is. Perhaps she had always suspected him or, if not, was she so wrapped in denial, so desperate to find Lysaght, that she lost what poor judgment she had? Now, as he sits on her bed, she viscerally realises (p. 155) that his small hands, his smell, his obesity, his blubbery lips, that voice, add up to something foul:

> She knows the girls are dead. There is something that states it in the room, in the hoarse breathing, in the sweat that for a moment touches the side of her

face, in the way he talks. The dark is oppressive with their deaths, cloying, threatening to turn odorous.

The end

After 'the act' he behaves out of the ordinary, unexpectedly. The previous girls hadn't brought out in him the need to distract with other things so why should this one? Why, a friendship has ended, that is all, nothing to worry about. But then he loses his appetite, sits and mopes, music un-played, *Daily Telegraph* unread. A visit to a stately home does some good, 'well it does you good to get out and about sometimes' and chancing into conversation with a lady, the moroseness goes and he gets his appetite back albeit temporarily. And then the Miss Calligary visits begin and he mentally unravels.

Why, he querulously asks, has *he* been picked out for attention by this black woman. Why is he being persecuted? Suspecting that he may be going insane, he decides to check this out. He reads:

> Delusional insanity is preceded by either maniacal or melancholic symptoms, and is not necessarily accompanied by any failure of the reasoning capacity. In the early stage the patient is introspective and uncommunicative, rarely telling his thoughts but brooding and worrying over them in secret. After this stage has lasted for a longer or shorter time the delusions become fixed and are generally of a disagreeable kind.
> (Trevor, 1995: 190)

And then, the penny drops! None of this has happened! The Calligary guilt stuff is some kind of mirage, the Irish girl has entranced him, thrown him into a spin, that's what they do those Irish, they're like sprites! Yet why can't he remember her? If only he could he might then induct her into his pantheon of 'the others' neatly tucked up, comfortably asleep. And then a suppressed thought steals into his mind unannounced stating that everything *is* real, that there is no mistake, that he has been seen, that things have been said.

If only chance hadn't brought the Irish girl into contact with the religious lunatics there wouldn't be this 'black woman threatening his privacy, poking and grubbing, flashing her teeth and her jewels, trapping him with her gibberish'. What's that Irish girl told them? Why does this religious woman talk of death all the time? Whose death? Now he knows why he can't remember the Irish girl's name. It's because she's alive, living proof of a reality beyond his consciousness, an insult to his designation of murder as 'ending a friendship'.

His death is witnessed by a cat. Actually the cat's not bothered, preoccupied as it is with a nearby saucepan of milk. It's a scavenger cat that may still crave the ordinariness of domesticity, just like Hilditch. As for Felicia, she becomes (p. 204) one of those girls:

on the run from a mess, or just wanting things to be different. Mysteries they're called when they are noticed on their journey; and in cities, or towns large enough to have trade in girls, the doors of Rovers and Volkswagens and Toyotas open to take them in. They try out the doorways of shops. There's a first time for everything they say, settling into this open air accommodation. Missing persons for a while, they then acquire a new identity. Riff-raff they're called now.

But that's not all. Remembering Hilditch, Felicia contemplates (p. 212) how: 'Lost within a man who murdered there was a soul like any other soul, purity itself it surely must have been.'

It's surely stretching things to see Hilditch as a victim, someone whom we might commiserate or sympathise with. But this is Trevor's take on deliverance, what Gerard Carruthers (2005: 117) calls: 'the creation of a particular ironic sympathy'. By weaving together loneliness, belonging, disengagement, and chance, by plotting histories on the reminiscences of Felicia and Hilditch, he forces an understanding of both characters' place in the scheme of things. He dies because she lives: chance has done its duty. She (p. 207) knows this and is not about to let go of destiny: So do her thoughts turn to how: 'the innocence that once was hers is now, with time, a foolishness, yet it is not disowned, and that same lost person is valued for leading her to where she is.' So this is what to expect from life's journey. Survival, as a first step, then the hard slog of working out where contentment is holed up. Felicia has found a liberty of sorts, free from life's baser constraints. Trevor imparts the following benediction: 'Walking through another morning, fine after a wet night, she accepts without bewilderment the serenity that possesses her, and celebrates its fresh new presence.' It's still awfully hard not to feel sorry for her, though.

Films

Atom Egoyan's (1999) film starring Bob Hoskins is very good. Faithful to the novel it misses some of its cultural and political tensions. But it captures well Felicia's sense of abandonment as she searches for her lover and Hoskins turns in a chilling, nuanced, performance as Mr Hilditch. Cinema is a different medium of course and Egoyan makes telling use of Hilditch's mother fixation when he shows him watching them together on old film. The point made, more clinically than in the book, is that madness originates in early, abusive, relationships and not in the here and now.

Both in the movie and the novel, 'English society' is depicted as cohesive only when viewed at 'the edges', for example, in the solidarity of homelessness or in Miss Calligary's 'gathering in' groups. The mainstream alternatively is a landscape of industrial and private ambition. As Felicia stops to buy a stale sausage role, Trevor describes the scene (pp. 101–2).

Already, hours ago, the homeless of this town have found night time resting places – in doorways, and underground passages left open in error, in abandoned vehicles, in the derelict gardens of demolished houses. As maggots make their way into cracks in masonry, so the people of the streets have crept into one-night homes in graveyards and on building sites, in alleyways and courtyards, making walls of dustbins pulled close together, and roofs of whatever lies nearby. Some have crawled up scaffolding to find a corner near the tarpaulin that protects an untiled expanse. Other have settled down in cardboard cartons that once contained dishwashers and refrigerators.

This is 'desolation row', straight from a Dickensian or other eighteenth- or nineteenth-century city underworld. And yet some of those she meets, for example George and Lena, are good people, kind and willing to share with her what little they've got. Like Felicia, they too will move on, drifting from the mainstream. Perhaps England's wasteland is where monsters are made, not born, that from alienation, rejection and repression comes evil. Well, yes, but then what of Hilditch's mother, the implication that either maternal upbringing (or genes) have done their unholy work? Or perhaps Mrs Hilditch is that familiar figure seen wandering through psychiatry's history, the female who brings evil in her wake, the epitome of male projection.

References

Carruthers, G (2005) Fictions of belonging. In BW Shaffer (ed), *The British and Irish Novel* (pp 112–27). London: Blackwell.

Del Rio Alvaro, C (2007) William Trevor's *Felicia's Journey*: Inherited dissent or fresh departure from tradition. *Estudios Irlandeses, 2,* 1–13.

Doyle, R (1987) *The Commitments*. Dublin: King Farouk Press.

Doyle, R (1991) *The Van*. London: Secker & Warburg.

Duguid, L (2002) Before it becomes literature. In Z Leader (ed), *On Modern British Fiction* (pp 284–303). Oxford: Oxford University Press.

Egoyan, A (1999) *Felicia's Journey* [film]. Hollywood: Warner Brothers.

Fuchs, C (2008) *Felicia's Journey*. Available online at: http://popmatters.com/film/felicias-journey.html

Gibbons, L (1996) *Transformations in Irish Culture*. Cork: Cork University Press.

Harris, T (1988) *Silence of the Lambs*. London: St Martin's Press.

Heaney, S (1995) Nobel Prize Lecture, Stockholm. Available online at: http://nobelprize.org/nobel_prizes/literature/laureates/1995/heaney-lecture.html

Jordan, N (1983) *The Dream of the Beast*. London: Chatto & Windus.

Jordan, N (2005) *Shade*. London: John Murray.

Kubrick, S (1980) *The Shining* [film]. Hollywood: Warner Bros.

MacKenna, D (1999) *William Trevor: The writer and his work*. Dublin: New Island.

McCabe, P (1992) *The Butcher Boy*. London: Picador.

St Peter, C (2002) Consuming pleasures: 'Felicia's Journey' in fiction and film. *Colby Quarterly, 38* (3), 329–39.

Trevor, W (1995) *Felicia's Journey*. London: Penguin.

CHAPTER 9

MACBETH

Did you ever have the feeling that you wanted to go,
But still have the feeling that you wanted to stay?
(Jimmy 'Schnozzola' Durante)

Introduction: the Machiavel

In Elizabethan theatre there flits, in and about its plays, a chameleon called the Machiavel. 'He' appears, famously, in Christopher Marlow's *Tamburlaine* as well as his *Jew of Malta*: a stock character that ingenuously dissembles and manipulates but, when over-extending itself, politically, socially or morally, typically comes a cropper. The type comes from Nicollo Machiavelli's *The Prince* (1961) where morality yields to circumstance, and where war is defensible in the acquisition of power and territory. And whilst it is better that a Prince attract love *and* fear, where he cannot have both, then it's preferable that he elicit fear. Elizabethans dreaded the disturbances such sentiments bring and audiences would have recoiled at the Machiavel and his equivocations no matter how flimsily drawn the character.

In earlier plays, Shakespeare had yet to abandon the thematic rules of Elizabethan theatre and so the Machiavel inhabited his work albeit less so as he kept writing. This is because what Shakespeare begins to do – moving on from *Richard III* to, especially, *Macbeth* is embellish stereotypical evil with greater emotional and psychological depth. Indeed, his depiction of history, comedy and tragedy races ahead of his contemporaries, both in complexity and breath.

Whereas in *Richard III,* the Machiavel appears in a pantomimic (Vice) style that is sinister and at times farcical, in *Macbeth* the full-bodied exchanges between Macbeth and his wife are the foreground to inner dialogues that reveal murderous instincts and self-recrimination. In this play, the Machiavel persists but as a shared duplicity as, for instance, when Lady Macbeth chides her husband:

To look like the innocent flower,
But be the serpent under't.
    (Act I, sc v)

Both *Macbeth* and *Richard III* sustain the proposition that when human will obtains free reign, it *diminishes* freedom. In other words, civilisation's mainstay is restraint: impeding the will profits the general good for even if, as individuals, we lose out materially, we still accrue moral and psychological profit. The Machiavel represents loss of constraint, a sprite that casts spells that dislocate integrity, will and good intentions.

Cost-benefit analysis

As mental health students, you may wish to compare this view (of restraint) with the theories of someone like Carl Rogers (2003) whose work you will be familiar with. Propounding a modish version of 'to thine own self be true', Rogers preached a concept of self-attainment achievable via forms of counselling that down-played how 'actualisation' might affect the general good. Even a cursory reading of Macbeth's terror as he oscillates between action and guilt damns 'actualisation' and the supposed primacy of 'self'. Macbeth knows that to assassinate a King is to tear society apart, that violating (the) divinity (of kings) exposes the world to devilish horrors. But he is driven beyond reason and when he falters, there is his wife to spur him on: she is the 'other', the shadow (this volume, Chapter 10) within his unconscious, an archetypal masculinity to which he is guiltily bound. The gulf is between individual ascendancy and universal welfare and its narrative base is the battle between reason and emotion, ambition and pity.

Ancient wisdoms

Ancient philosophers, for example Socrates, argued that reason governs choices between right and wrong, that we cannot do wrong knowing it to be such. Yet, when tempted, how many of us give way knowing that we shouldn't, reason overcome by desire, judgement falling before passion. It's an intricate combination, emotion and reason, and, in this play, its communication is less about: 'uncovering the crime to others than with the uncovering of the criminal to himself' (Hunter, 1967: 7). Our becoming privy to Macbeth's thought moves the drama onto a new and complex plane. When Richard exclaims: 'I am determined to prove a villain', we recognise this as less a sign of strength and more the Machiavel's desire to celebrate human discomfort. There is more to *Richard III* than this, of course, but with *Macbeth* matters penetrate to a denser level: we get *inside* Macbeth's imagination, watch him succumb to recrimination and terror. It reminds you of Kafka (this volume, Chapter 7) whose:

> distinctive ability as a writer ... was to render visible, in symbolic form, the way this type of thinking operates. He lays bare the state of mind, the motivation, the attitudes on which its interpretation of the world is based.
> (Thorlby, 1972: 89)

As did Shakespeare, opening up awareness in symbolic as well as in acutely human terms. For instance, an ordinary mortal, hearing the witch's predictions, would have straightaway inquired into their meaning: but Macbeth's brain over-leaps the here-and-now speculating on what's in it for him. The witches appeal to what he *wants* to hear (Johnston, 2007): they don't put ideas (of murder) *into* his head; King Duncan isn't even mentioned and why need he be when he permeates Macbeth's thinking already.

This is a play of extraordinary intimacy. The murder which lies at its heart is represented to us through Macbeth's consciousness of it, both before and after and not by the murder itself. It's as though the idea of murder is worse than the thing itself. Unlike Richard III who 'plays to the galleries', this protagonist comments on his own thoughts before us, drawing us in like mental osmosis. Equally, especially before the deed, are we made party to the Macbeths' powerful intimacy with each other and how they communicate their reliance on each other, particularly his dependence on her.

So what's Macbeth about?

It's straightforward really. The play takes place mostly in Scotland and, as it begins, Duncan reigns as a 'sweet-natured' King. Returning from victorious battles against invading armies, Macbeth and Banquo (two of Duncan's Generals) encounter three witches. The witches predict, improbably, that Macbeth will become Thane (Lord) of Cawdor (there is already a Lord of Cawdor) and eventually King of Scotland. Banquo will not become King, say the hags, but will sire a line of Kings.

Following this encounter, the generals are met by King Duncan's men who tell them that Macbeth is now Thane of Cawdor, the previous incumbent facing imminent execution for treason. Stunned, Macbeth turns to Banquo:

Macbeth:
Do you not hope your children shall be Kings,
When those that gave the Thane of Cawdor to me
Promised no less to them?

Banquo:
That, trusted home,
Might yet enkindle you unto the crown,
Besides the Thane of Cawdor. But 'tis strange:
And oftentimes, to win us to our harm,
The instruments of darkness tell us truths,
Win us with honest trifles, to betray's
In deepest consequence.

Macbeth: [aside]
Two truths are told,
As happy prologues to the swelling act
Of the imperial theme …
This supernatural soliciting
Cannot be ill, cannot be good. If ill,
Why hath it given me earnest of success
Commencing in a truth? I am Thane of Cawdor.
If good, why do I yield to that suggestion
Whose horrid image doth unfix my hair,
And make my seated heart knock at my ribs,
Against the use of nature? Present fears
Are less than horrible imaginings.
My thought, whose murder yet is but fantastical,
Shakes so my single state of man that function
Is smothered in surmise, and nothing is
But what is not.
    (Act I, sc iii)

Imagination, murder, hesitation, guilt, retribution, contradiction, gender, equivocation: these will be the themes of this play: incessantly.

    A perturbed Macbeth invites Duncan to sup at his castle forewarning his Lady that the King is on his way as well as apprising her of the witchs' predictions. She however has intuited her husband's thoughts and is already bent on regicide with seeming equanimity. Pooh-poohing her husband's misgivings she urges murder *that very night,* her intention being to ply Duncan's bodyguards with drink so that:

when in swinish sleep
Their drenched natures lie, as in a death,
What cannot you and I perform upon
The unguarded Duncan? What not put upon
His spongy officers, who shall bear the guilt
Of our great quell?
    (Act I, sc vii)

The deed accomplished, the body discovered, alarms sounded, Macbeth crashes into the King's chamber and, feigning outrage at his murder, kills the two guards. Duncan's sons, fearing for their lives, flee to England and Ireland. Macbeth, cognizant that Banquo's heirs will be Kings, pays assassins to kill Banquo and his son. But when they fail to kill the boy Macbeth's mire of mental indecision deepens. Hosting a ceilidh for the Scottish nobility he is visited by Banquo's ghost and his audible consternation (despite Lady Macbeth's reassurances) causes the nobles to suspect him.

Macbeth again visits the witches who reassure him with new but ever more odd-sounding predictions. He cannot, they tell him, be killed by man of woman born and until Birnam Wood comes to his castle at Dunsinane, he will be safe. Well, you can't buck promises like that: a wood doesn't move and all men are from women born! It looks like Macbeth is home and dry. Nevertheless, the doubts, torments, rages persist and when Macduff joins King Duncan's sons abroad, Macbeth orders his family wiped out. By now he is 'gorging on blood' as:

> Each new morn
> New widows howl, new orphans cry, new sorrows
> Strike heaven on the face, that it resounds
> As if it felt with Scotland and yell'd out
> Like syllable of dolour.
> (Act IV, sc iii)

Descending into hopelessness, Macbeth still relates believably to his surroundings, especially as threats mount up against him. Conversely, Lady Macbeth now wanders the castle battlements, trying to wash off blood that somehow won't wash off. Learning of his wife's problems, Macbeth (Act V, sc iii) charges his doctor:

> Canst thou not minister to a mind diseased,
> Pluck from the memory a rooted sorrow,
> Raze out the written troubles of the brain,
> And with some sweet oblivious antidote
> Cleanse the stuffed bosom of that perilous stuff
> Which weighs upon the heart?

When the doctor says she must (emotionally) fend for herself, Macbeth explodes, 'Throw physic to the dogs! I'll none of it.' It's an exchange that implies that the Lady is profoundly depressed, wracked with guilt. Macbeth had hoped for a potion to lighten her load but there *is* no such medicine: in effect, Mr and Mrs Macbeth, 'having made their bed must now lie on it'. Look at the lines (above): there comes a 'perilous stuff' from a 'stuffed bosom', a 'rooted sorrow' made worse by the workings of the brain. Apart from being a brilliant synthesis of reason and emotion what else does it suggest? Is there, for instance, a lost child somewhere in the play? Macduff's anguished cry: 'He has no children' doesn't mean that the Macbeths have never had a child though this might be the case. But could childlessness drive them to state terrorism and destruction? Possibly: but whereof the origins of this child? Is it mythic or real, imagined or contrived? (See, in this instance, the movie *Who's Afraid of Virginia Wolf* (Nichols, 1966) where a 'phantom child' inducts misery, subterfuge and, ultimately, tragedy into a marriage.) David Willbern (1993) points out that *Macbeth* takes place in a world where clear distinctions like man/woman, night/day, fair/foul, real/ imagined, are blurred. So what price *this* child? Is it or has it ever been real? Or is it, as psychoanalysis would suggest, a metaphor that lies beyond the Macbeths' comprehension, or us who watch them? Lady Macbeth, in a classic example of reaction formation, converts a putative maternal love into one of loathing and murderous design: for are not her antinatal rages a denial of what is maternally plausible? Or, maybe, as John Bayley (1981) mentions, Macbeth is the child and when he resists her admonishments she will turn her milk to gall and feed him with it.

This is where logic dissolves and imagination runs riot. Macbeth kills children, literally, and with Banquo he kills the possibility of their birth. With his wife's suicide, Macbeth's mood plummets and when Dunsinane Wood comes into view (as hand-held branches used as military camouflage) he knows the jig is up. But not yet: like Richard, Macbeth will fight to the end and, as battle commences, a cruel equivocation takes place when Macduff tells him that he was 'untimely ripped from his mother's womb'. What splendid duplicity is this! How easy it is to imagine him hysterically plunging towards Macduff's sword. And now Malcolm is King – declaring benevolence towards all men and nations, of course – and peace returns to the Scots or, more so, Kingship, until the next Richard or Macbeth crawls from the undergrowth.

Macbeth had entered the play as a War Lord, chest out, up for anything (in Antony Sher's production, he comes on stage carried shoulder high to the sounds of victorious football chants) and it was in this mood that he received the witches' first predictions and where, instantly, his head reeled with such fantastical 'what ifs' that the hair stood on his head. It's an intriguing idea that guilt kicks in *before* the evil act. So that when the murder is done it has already gone against his better judgement. However, in psychology, it has been argued that although we invariably think of behaviour as a consequence of thought, for example, that we run because we are afraid, matters may be more complex than that. The contention of psychologist William James (1890) was that we are afraid because we are running. Called the 'James-Lange Theory', it asserts that behaviour runs in feedback loops, that if we perceive something (an accelerating pulse for instance) as evidence of an imminent heart attack, this perception will drive up further physical changes which in turn add to the initial belief. Thus are Macbeth's vile activities self-confirmation of his inherent malevolence and which propels all the more his descent into self-obfuscation and misery and where release will only come, as for Richard, in battle and death.

A gender bender?

Gender pervades *Macbeth*. At first we wonder if the witches are psychological projections of Macbeth's fears. Although insofar as Banquo also sees them we may suppose they are real enough albeit who or what can they be? Are they

117

indeed women? They call each other 'sister' so it would seem so. Yet, on meeting them (Act I, sc iii), Banquo calls out:

> What are these,
> So withered and so wild in their attire,
> That look not like the inhabitants o' the earth,
> And yet are on't? Live you? ...
> You should be women;
> And yet your beards forbid me to interpret
> That you are so.

Are they a remembrance of 'the Fall', a collegiate Eve presaging man's spiritual ruin? They foreshadow what will come, which is not to say that they instigate it. Theirs is a commencement of contradiction, of fair *and* foul, male and female, unsettlement. At the end of Act IV, when news breaks of the slaughter of Macduff's family, Malcolm provokes Macduff to: 'Dispute it like a man' to which Macduff replies: 'I shall do so; But I must also feel it as a man.'

Macbeth is about manliness. Hearing of the King's impending visit, Lady Macbeth resolves to kill him: she aches for the Crown but has a problem, a husband whose nature: 'is too full o' the milk of human-kindness To catch the nearest way.' She knows he wants the spoils, but she knows better his reluctance to do the dirty in order to get them. So, psychotic like, she broadcasts her thoughts to him.

> Hie thee hither
> That I may pour my sprits in thine ear,
> And chastise with the valour of my tongue
> All that impedes thee from the golden round.
>   (Act I, sc v)

This feels odd because *he* is the King's champion, *he* is the victorious warrior who laughed at fear in the killing fields. Did not one of his sergeant's describe: 'His brandish'd steel, Which smoked with bloody execution' and that, confronting an enemy: 'he unseam'd him from the nave to the chaps, and fix'd his head upon our battlements.'

But murder is different, its call not to 'the colours' but to sating desires whose consequences Macbeth dreads. So, in the play's most terrifying passage (Act I, sc v), it is she who heralds murder.

> The raven himself is hoarse
> That croaks the fatal entrance of Duncan
> Under my battlements. Come, you spirits
> That tend on mortal thoughts, unsex me here,
> And fill me, from the crown to the toe, top-full

Of direst cruelty! Make thick my blood,
Stop up the access and passage to remorse,
That no compunctious visitings of nature
Shake my fell purpose, nor keep peace between
The effect and it! Come to my woman's breasts,
And take my milk for gall, you murdering ministers,
Wherever in your sightless substances
You wait on nature's mischief! Come, thick night,
And pall thee in the dunnest smoke of hell,
That my keen knife see not the wound it makes,
Nor heaven peep through the blanket of the dark,
To cry 'Hold, hold!'

When Macbeth mentions the King's departure the next day, she declares differently and when this startles him she admonishes:

Your face, my thane, is as a book where men
May read strange matters. To beguile the time,
Look like the time; bear welcome in your eye,
Your hand, your tongue: look like the innocent flower,
But be the serpent under't. He that's coming
Must be provided for.

Richard himself could hardly match this bare-faced trickery and so sinister is its affect that Macbeth says they will talk no more of it. Later, peeved at her jibes, he snaps: 'I dare do all that may become a man; Who dares do more is none.' And still she piles it on telling him that when he dared do it he was a man and would be again if he'd just stop this nonsense! Notice the accusatory allusion to *milk* – how he is stuffed with it – and when she snarls that, rather than break a promise to *him,* she would pluck her nipple from the smiling face of a suckling infant and bash its brains out, he damns her fit to bear male children only. Yet within a minute he agrees to do the deed. If 'all the world's a stage', its men and women merely players, then life is a charade, a thought that hasn't escaped psychologists and sociologists (Freud, 1968; Berne, 1966; Goffman, 1968) but it doesn't make life less liveable. Rather does it render identity ambiguous so that it must/needs present itself in alternative ways. (See *As You Like It* where Shakespeare again plays with ambivalence, homoeroticism and gender switching.)

A Freudian Macbeth

In a post-Freudian world of imagery, metaphor (and pessimism) we are accustomed to a 'reality' driven by repression and denial. Having just killed Duncan (Act II, sc iii), Macbeth declares;

> Had I but died an hour before this chance
> I had lived a blessed time; for from this instant
> There's nothing serious in mortality.
> All is but toys, renown and grace is dead,
> The wine of life is drawn, and the mere lees
> Is left this vault to brag of.

In truth, he knew this the moment he met the witches and since when everything has been topsy turvy. When he met them they were both of the earth and not, tantalisingly short on information yet quick to seize the (dis)temper of *his* mind. And on it goes. When he panics before Banquo's ghost, Lady Macbeth tries to calm him, at one point asking if he really is a man and when he replies (whimsically) that he must be since he has dared look upon a ghost, she compares him to old women who tell stories by the fire.

Freud began reading Shakespeare aged eight and continued to do so throughout his life (and was ever ready to filch appropriate quotes when needed!). In fact, his standing as a Shakespearean student is considerable. Some productions owe him a great deal – for example, Olivier's *Hamlet* with its stress on father-son relationships and the Oedipal complex. Likewise Antony Sher's depiction of Richard III as a sexual predator, a male garlanded in arachnid's clothing. That said, Shakespeare scholar Harold Bloom insists that we typically link Shakespeare and Freud the wrong way around, that Freudian psychology is *heir* to Shakespeare, it is *Shakespeare* who formulates 'neurosis' to which Freud attaches a scientific terminology. Indeed, what are Freud's efforts at analysing Shakespeare other than the Oedipal resentment of a more powerful literary/historical figure!

Intriguingly, Freud doesn't over-analyse *Macbeth*. Unsurprisingly, he dwells on fathers and sons in respect of the killings and, as well, he identifies Macbeth's rage as born of his (apparent) inability to procreate: Banquo shall have sons but not Macbeth:

> If one surveys the whole play … one sees that it is sown with references to the father–children relation. The murder of the kindly Duncan is little else but patricide; in Banquo's case, Macbeth kills the father whilst the son escapes him; and in Macduff's, he kills the children because the father has fled from him. A bloody child, and then a crowned one, are shown him by the witches in the apparition scene; the armed head which is seen earlier is no doubt Macbeth himself.
> (Freud, 1968: 134)

Freud's psychological touch is light, his literary insights more evenly worked through. He observes how authorial interference with narrative plausibility is fine when it brings greater insights (to audiences) and he mentions the meeting between Richard and Anne, in *Richard III*, as a case in point. It *is* odd, he says, how she capitulates so quickly but, in the balance, it heightens admiration (and unease) at Richard's sexual prowess. It shows how Shakespeare constructs encounters from which improbable relationships take root and grow. What does she see in him? How blind can a person be? True: but how many times has this been asked of how many others? Freud also mentions the unlikelihood of Lady Macbeth's progress, one minute homicidally egging her husband on, the next disclaiming suicidal impulses and obsessive-compulsive behaviour. In this, Shakespeare positions fear/apprehension next to anxiety/obsession demonstrating how obsessions block anxiety and anticipatory existential destruction. Compulsive obsessions use up the time between their execution and death and that's their point, the human difficulty of contemplating the inevitable.

Yet, whilst her distress is sudden, earlier events suggest vulnerability: 'These deeds must not be thought After these ways; so, it will make us mad' (as for her it does). Or earlier still, when she remarks that had Duncan not resembled her father, she would have done for him then and there. Actually, you have to wonder why she *didn't* kill Duncan herself. That he reminded her of her Dad may be a self-serving conceit or perhaps things had just moved too quickly with no time to think, to detach herself from the rush of events. Within a week (of the action of the play) there has occurred mass murder, torrential storms, shipwrecks, betrayal, obsessive anxiety, supernatural events, depression, suicide, *inertia*: 'I am in blood Stepped in so far, that, should I wade no more, Returning were as tedious as go o'er' (Act III, sc iv).

Inertia: and, as well, timelessness. Recall Macbeth's letter to his wife announcing the imminent arrival of Duncan and which transports her 'beyond this ignorant present' such that she feels 'the future in an instant'. Between that instant, and tomorrow, Duncan will die. In this, the play is cast in a Freudian time-warp of past and present converging in a moment. But concerned that Macbeth will reveal what's afoot in the moment, she orders him to conceal his darker desires: think only, she says, about 'our nights and days to come'. We all of us at times lock into moments whose meaning lies in fantasy whether future or past. Fantasy? In this case maybe not, because they both finally go mad, she psychotically, whilst he, resolved to go down in blood, likens himself to a chained beast: 'They have tied me to a stake; I cannot fly But, bear like, I must fight the course.' At which point, Lady Macbeth loses her grip: even the oceans, she wails, can't wash the blood off and at the end she appears to kill herself. No doubt, like me, some of you thought that *she* would have lasted the course with Macbeth collapsing into some fugue state, wandering off to death, leaving her to clean up the mess.

A multiple personality?

However, playing Mr & Mrs misses the point about the Macbeths. It's hard, actually, to conceive of them separately and it's only when they are together, in madness or death, that they – and the play – hold together. Macbeth's angst occurs before Duncan's murder but continues after the murder in *her*. Freud (1968: 137) notes how they endlessly go over the possible reactions to the crime: 'like two disunited parts of a single psychical individuality.'

We know that killing *per se* is not what ailed Macbeth but 'that in killing Duncan he would be violating every rule that holds his community together' (Johnston, 2007), and that this would return to haunt him. In Act I, sc vii Macbeth states:

> But in these cases
> We still have judgement here; that we but teach
> Bloody instructions, which, being taught, return
> To plague the inventor. This even-handed justice
> Commends the ingredients of our poisoned chalice
> To our own lips.

Still, he *wants* to be king: *she* wants him King and her goading is an itch that he cannot scratch. 'I have no spur To prick the sides of my intent, but only Vaulting ambition, which o'er-leaps itself And falls on the other' which means: I am born to rule, but unlikely to reign. Both are imperious but lack the enabling interest (in others) that makes worthy rule possible. Macbeth has nobility and is capable of chivalrous impulses but neither of them live by these. Others have judged them less harshly:

> They have no separate ambitions. They support and love one another. They suffer together. And if, as time goes on, they drift a little apart, they are no vulgar souls, to be alienated and recriminate when they experience the fruitlessness of their ambition. They remain to the end tragic, even grand.
> (Bradley, 1905: 104)

And they perish separately: not for them the sweet mockery of expiring in each others arms!

Feasibly, Lady Macbeth doesn't understand her husband – witness the losses of temper, the goading, the sarcasm. But her reactions are less about him as about her understanding his need of her as agent provocateur, shoring up his darker ego. He has seemed the more human with his doubts and hesitancies. Yet does he accede to her demands surprisingly quickly. Marriage has honed his ambition, clothed him in expectations albeit without quashing his tendency to ruminate on the wrath of God. If, as Lady Macbeth believes, these fears are the superficial ranting of nervous debility, then they would lapse into hysteria. But they are more than this: his uncertainties remind us of his once strong moral imperative as well as the irreconcilability of conscience with murder and how a smothered conscious begets destruction and death as its end point.

Homicidal

Macbeth has been called a tragedy of ambition, and a tragedy of terror. This is not true. There is only one theme in Macbeth: murder. History has been reduced to its form, to one image and one division: those who kill and those who are killed.

(Kott, 1967: 69–70)

This is a play that is 'sticky and thick' with blood and when (influenced by Kott) Roman Polanski filmed it, he flooded the screen in maroon. This alarmed his co-writer, Ken Tynan, until Polanski informed him that, having witnessed the aftermath of (his wife) Sharon Tate's murder by the Charles Manson gang, he knew what murder *looked* like. So does Lady Macbeth cry: 'Who would have thought the old man to have so Much blood in him?' And returning to the theme of gender Willbern (1993: 111) remarks: 'To be a man, in this tragedy's central terms, means to be bloody or bloodied. Wounds are the mark of manliness.' Todd London (1998: 64) sees it in similar terms:

Macbeth is the ur-weird play [ur = original], where destiny and sorcery, prophecy and madness impregnate one another, and everything born of their couplings dies, until bodies and babies and words pile together in a bizarre imagistic bloodbath. Certainly the Macbeths would be at home in Sarajevo or Rwanda.

It *is* about murder: that's true, but not completely so. Kott locates Shakespeare in a mid-twentieth century reeling from fascism and especially the Holocaust – which Kott had experienced – as well as the general brutality of war and slaughter. People with such experiences (Freud was stained by the horrors of the 1914–18 War and anti-Semitism) are ingrained with pessimism. Samuel Beckett (1959) captures this in his famous opening line in *Waiting for Godot*: 'Nothing to be done.' It was to Beckett that R.D. Laing turned in describing madness from the despair and alienation of his patient's stories. Echoing Beckett, Laing (1960: 42) mused: 'One enters a world in which there is no contradictory sense of the self in its "health and validity" to mitigate the despair, terror, and boredom of existence.'

When Peter Brook filmed *King Lear* (starring Paul Scofield) he too saw it in the 'stripped down' fashion of Kott's ideas and Becket's prose, its bloodless characterisation, its emptied out, wasteland, finish a worthy epitaph to twentieth century totalitarianism. Never was the horror more realised than in the claim: 'I was only obeying orders', the contention that one is a small cog in a much larger wheel. Hannah Arendt (1963) talks of 'the banality of evil', the nucleus of evil that beats within tedium and bureaucratisation. The point is well made by Leonard Cohen (1964; 78) in his poem:

All There Is To Know About Adolph Eichmann

Eyes:	Medium
Hair:	Medium
Weight:	Medium
Height:	Medium
Distinguishing features:	None
Number of Fingers:	Ten
Intelligence:	Medium
What Did You Expect?	
Talons?	
Oversize Incisors?	
Green Saliva?	
Madness?	

Arendt's observations were based on the Eichmann trial with the Holocaust, as she saw it, a product of ordinariness in the sense of the mechanics of 'solving a problem'. It's a controversial idea dependent on the belief that Eichmann (and his ilk) were governed by an anti-Semitism so ingrained that it went beyond moral consideration or judgement. It is also a contention that goes against the received wisdom of 'the killer' as somehow monstrous, larger than life, mad. That said, there is, in fact, ample evidence of gratuitous torture and killing not constrained by the numbers involved or notions of the mechanics of problem solving (see James, 2001 for an excellent résumé on this question).

And yet the Macbeths become *interesting people*. How can this be? At the end, each day bringing newer and greater atrocities, it's hard to understand our fascination with this couple or wanting to know more about them. Perhaps the answer lies nearer to our own time, to the commonality of tyranny across cultures and countries as in Pol Pot, Milosevic or Mugabe. As we watch the slaughter on our TV screens we would reel in disgust were the perpetrators represented as *interesting*. That said, some recent films show a (deplorable) tendency towards presenting individual Nazis as human and/or complex, providing them with roles that extirpate the horror they wrought. Examples are Polanski's *The Pianist* (2002), Paul Verhoeven's *Black Book* (2006) and Bryan Singer's *Valkyrie* (2008), all of which ascribe variants of nobility to Nazi characters. Most notably, the film *The Reader*, in which Kate Winslet portrays a Nazi camp guard, was described by the head of the New York Simon Wiesenthal Centre as 'one of a series of recent Hollywood films that were guilty of holocaust revisionism' (Shipman, 2009). Not everyone agreed with this but the concerns are real enough and may cause some future pause for thought.

Macbeth kicks because whilst it doesn't let up on its protagonists' evil, despite their invocations of horror and butchery, it deals with these in terms of their consciousness. The evil which men and women have wrought throughout humanity are awful to *behold* and neither of the Macbeths spare us the agonies of their ruminations on their bloody deeds. It's as if they've become stuck in the blood so that there can be no way to turn, certainly no going back. There lacks even an appeal to God whose cosmos they have wrecked with their almost helpless malice. The belief in the supernatural has helped the story to advance psychologically because it darkens all the more the sense of what has been violated. It hasn't in fact been necessary to show us Duncan's murder since it is incidental to the recognition of a usurper dissecting his consciousness before us.

Supernatural

Today's interpretations of *Macbeth* are psychological, for instance, depicting Banquo's ghost as a *projection* of Macbeth's guilt. The problem with this though is that, in *Macbeth,* the supernatural is believed in and not just by the poor or uneducated. Wealthy, even scholarly, Elizabethans were also fearful of unworldly forces when thwarted. *Macbeth* was written in 1606, about six years before ten people were hanged at Lancaster for 'murdering' seventeen others through witchcraft. Some of the Lancastrian witches confessed their guilt without pressure, suggesting that they may have been deluded.

> The ... witches were deformed, retarded, epileptic, facially disfigured, or, like the widow Chattox, then in her eighties, "a very old withered spent and decreped creature, her sight almost gone ... her lippes ever chattering ... but no man knew what", in the words of one contemporary account.
> (Vallely, 1998: 14)

Notice the similarity in description of the widow Chattox and Shakespeare's witches: decrepit, withered, blind, chattering. Witchcraft, at the time, was a hot political potato and governments strove to assure the public that they were 'doing something about it'. Witch-finding was the 'at-risk register' of its generation and witch sacrifices were perpetrated by local political bigwigs anxious to please James I of England whose interest in witchcraft was deep-seated. He had written *the* book on the subject – and he would have seen *Macbeth*: Shakespeare certainly had him in mind when he wrote it.

Equivocation

The witches epitomise equivocation. *Macbeth* was staged at the time of the Gunpowder Plot (1605) when Catholic clerics declared it acceptable for plotters to equivocate under questioning so as to save themselves. Therefore, the political and moral dangers of slipperiness were uppermost in people's minds and not least King James's against whom the audacious plot was directed. Shakespeare pounces on this from the first (Act I, sc III) when Banquo exclaims:

> But 'tis strange,
> And oftentimes, to win us to our harm,
> The instruments of darkness tell us truths,
> Win us with honest trifles, to betray's
> In deepest consequence.

His is the conservative voice, the audiences' conduit to fear of terrorism and insurrection. The witches have 'appeared' swathed in dark and foul air. It is difficult to make them out. Nothing about them – their appearance at any rate – is clear other than they culture the unworldliness of the play. Macbeth's destruction stems from this, his failure to heed his moral inclinations, to allow his reason greater leeway over the phantasmagorical which gets to him every time. Hearing things, seeing things, imagining things; even in battle he is no rational killer, his (and Banquo's) recklessness, ('aimless ferocity') described 'As cannons overcharg'd with double cracks; So they doubly redoubled strokes upon the foe: Except they meant to bathe in reeking wounds' (Act I, sc ii).

If he could only attend to where 'present fears' might take him. But he wants *majesty*. It's as though he's caught between sleeping and waking, paralysed with indecision:

> Why do I yield to that suggestion
> Whose horrid image doth unfix my hair
> And make my seated heart knock at my ribs,
> Against the use of nature? Present fears
> Are less than horrible imaginings;
> My thought, whose murder yet is but fantastical,
> Shakes so my single state of man that function
> Is smother'd in surmise, and nothing is
> But what is not.
>   (Act I, sc iii)

His recriminative thought fires him into action whilst pulling him back from it. His is a brinkmanship where: 'thought jumps to action, action is overtaken by consequence, with a precipitate haste, as if it were all written breathlessly' (Irving & Marshall, 1922: 13). Like a gambler hunting 'the jackpot' so will just one more murder seize the time. But this can't be, because such acts profoundly affect others. Macbeth and his Lady sought domination proceeding from a universal principle of kingship but to achieve this they had to murder a King, a divine provocation, tempting transcendent disaster and you can smell their terror as they slide towards annihilation. Having murdered sleep Macbeth must act out his fantasies whilst awake. He is a psyche turned inside out obsessively doing what he would rather not and for whom the only rational act left – to go back – is beyond hope. But this is no morality play: what we see are 'present imaginings' clouded between wish and desire, spaces between acts and consequences, between thought and action, the space (of the play) is where people flounder, as we watch, knowing that they are us.

Films

Macbeth

Orson Welles's *Macbeth* (1948), starring himself, rejects naturalism for an adjusted text filmed against sets influenced by German Expressionism. Interestingly, the actors speak in Scottish accents but it is the use of striking images, especially shadows, that gives the film an edgy symbolism. In this movie evil reigns supreme, with goodness a pale, cowardly, distraction:

> Visually, the film is filled with distortions – vast foreground figures dwarfing those in the background, axe-blades and hands spread across the screen, shadows on rough walls or passing ominously over human figures.
>   (Jorgens, 1977: 151–2)

It's a rough-hewn film, mean, unsubtle, gothic. In part, the abstract, minimalist sets resulted from Welles, as usual, being strapped for cash. But as Macbeth, he dominates the action playing the role as if in a dream, appearing sometimes as if drunk or hypnotised, for example when murdering Duncan. In other words, this is a tyrant not just out of political control, but beyond psychological jurisdiction as well.

In this 1955 movie, *Joe Macbeth*, Paul Douglas plays Joe Macbeth with Sid James as Banky and Gregoire Asian as Duca, their boss. Philip Yordan, the writer, doesn't stretch the original too far but transfers it to hoodlum New York. The castle becomes a Gothic Lakeside villa – of the sort favoured by Mafiosi – and Banquo's appearance is treated as a tarot card-reading. The film's darkness, small interiors, and gangster violence give it an overall macabre character.

The Tragedy of Macbeth

Directed by Roman Polanski (1971) *The Tragedy of Macbeth* followed upon the murder of Polanski's wife (and others) by the Charles Manson Gang. The film thus acquired an air of sensation. It's an interesting question, the extent to which the murders influenced the movie. For example, in the play the murders take place off stage and many have used this mechanism to disturb the imagination. Polanski, however, shows murder in its awfulness, sparing us little.

Shot on location and with expensively made sets, the film recreates better than any the hustle and bustle of castle life. The two main players are physically attractive with Jon Finch's King consistent with the status of a young warrior. The actors were helped in that their longer speeches are delivered as 'voiceovers' and not directly to camera. But chiefly, it is the symbolic imagery behind Shakespeare's words that is brilliantly realised by clever cinematography aided by an edgy music score and this is what Polanski's direction may have been about.

Throne of Blood was directed by legendary Japanese director Akira Kurosawa in 1957 with Toshiro Mifune in the lead role. Harold Bloom, a major Shakespearean scholar, has called it the best film version and Peter Brook, perhaps the most intellectually gifted of British stage directors, calls it 'a masterpiece': neither are alone in this view.

The film moves – as it should – as sequences of symbolic tableau. Rosenthal (2000: 76) comments that: 'There is no poetry in *Throne of Blood*'s sparse dialogue, and little subtlety in its characterisation [the Lady Macbeth figure hardly speaks] but its pace, atmosphere and imagery are absolutely Shakespearean.' For instance, there is a riveting sequence where the Macbeths become lost in an eerie cobweb-maze where they meet with a 'witch' character whose white facial makeup comes from Japanese Noh theatre and the effect is as disturbing as it is disorientating. This is not a filmed play. Rather is it the one true translation of Shakespeare in filmic terms.

References

Arendt, H (1963) *Eichmann in Jerusalem*. London: Faber.

Bayley, J (1981) *Shakespeare and Tragedy*. London: Routledge & Kegan Paul.

Beckett, S (1959) *Waiting for Godot*. London: Faber & Faber.

Berne, E (1966) *Games People Play*. London: Andre Deutsch.

Bradley, AC (1905) *Shakespearian Tragedy: Lecture on Hamlet, Othello, King Lear, Macbeth* (2nd edn). London: Macmillan.

Cohen, L (1964) *Flowers for Hitler*. London: Jonathan Cape.

Durante, J (1942) *The Man Who Came to Dinner*[film]. (Dir. W. Keighley) Hollywood: Warner Bros.

Freud, S (1968) From some character-types met with in psycho-analytic work. In J Wain (ed), *Macbeth* (pp. 131–8). London: Macmillan.

Goffman, E (1968) *Asylums*. Harmondsworth: Penguin.

Hughes, K (1955) *Joe Macbeth* [film]. UK: Columbia Pictures.

Hunter, GK (1967) Introduction: *Macbeth*. Harmondsworth: Penguin.

Irving, H & Marshall, FA (1922) *The Works of William Shakespeare Vol. 11*. London: The Gresham Publishing Company.

James, C (2001) Hitler's unwilling exculpator. In *Reliable Essays: The best of Clive James* (pp 234–56). London: Picador.

James, W (1890) *The Principles of Psychology*. Mineola, NY: Dover Press.

Johnston, I (2007) Personal communication.

Jorgens, J (1977) *Shakespeare on Film*. London: Indiana University Press.

Kott, J (1967) *Shakespeare: Our contemporary* (2nd edn). London: Methuen.

Kurosawa, A (1957) *Throne of Blood* [film]. UK: BFI/Connoisseur Video.

Laing, RD (1960) *The Divided Self*. London: Tavistock.

London, T (1998) Shakespeare in a strange land. *American Theatre, 15* (6), 22–5, 63–6.

Machiavelli, N (1961) *The Prince*. Harmondsworth: Penguin Classics. [Original work published 1515]

Nichols, M (1966) *Who's Afraid of Virginia Woolf?* [film]. Hollywood: Warner Bros.

Polanski, R (1971) *The Tragedy of Macbeth* [film]. US: Columbia Tristar.

Polanski, R (2002) *The Pianist* [film]. Hollywood: Universal Pictures.

Rogers, CR (2003) *Client-Centered Therapy*. London: Constable.

Rosenthal, D (2000) *Shakespeare on Screen*. London: Hamlyn.

Shakespeare, W (1967) *Macbeth*. Harmondsworth: Penguin. [Original work published 1606]

Shipman, T (2009) Historian's war on Winslet. *The Sunday Telegraph*: 23.

Singer, B (2008) *Valkyrie* [film]. Hollywood: United Artists.

Thorlby, A (1972) *A Student's Guide to Kafka*. London: Heinemann Educational.

Vallely, P (1998) Spirit of the age: Toil and trouble on a black hill. *The Independent, 31* October, 14.

Verhoeven, P (2006) *Black Book* [film]. Netherlands: A Films.

Welles, O (1948) *Macbeth* [film]. UK: Second Sight Films.

Willbern, D (1993) Phantasmagorical Macbeth. In PL Rudnytsky (ed), *Transitional Objects and Potential Spaces* (pp 101–34). New York: Columbia University Press.

STEPPENWOLF

Now this be the Law of the Jungle as old and as true as the sky;
And the Wolf that shall keep it may prosper, but the Wolf that shall break it
must die.
   (Rudyard Kipling, *The Law of the Jungle*)

On the barren straits of the Russian steppes wanders a species of wolf – *Canis lupus campestris* – supposedly only listlessly connected to sociality and whose primary resolve is sniffing out morsels of food to stay alive. You may be surprised to learn that Harry Haller, a human being, is also a wolf of the Steppes. You might want to know how this can be. Well, it's because, like the wolf, the world holds little meaning or joy for him. He believes himself bereft of any capacity for social relevance; middle-class 'standards' revolt him. However, their comforts entice, and he can't deprive himself of the pleasures they bring. Like a house divided, Harry can't orient himself towards his fellows, an internal division he tries to conceal by distancing himself from humanity – and so avoiding the label 'schizoid'. But he knows that acting within convention is valued within liberal societies and that challenging this may invite derision. So, seeking love, but disdaining companionship, Harry becomes discontent, not infrequently contemplating suicide.

As students of psychiatry, we recognise this inclination to self-destruct only too well. There is much in the psychosocial literature that links states of *anomie* – Durkheim's (1989) concept of being adrift from society (even when in the midst of it) – and the tendency to dissolution that such states bring. Equally, if we peruse Brown and Harris's (1978) seminal study of depression, we find much that positively correlates anomie with social status, class, bad housing, humiliation and disenchantment. Yet, in studying Harry, the protagonist of Herman Hesse's novel *Steppenwolf,* we get a view of alienation *viscerally*, we feel his depression, its apprehension, dread and decay.

Preamble

Steppenwolf (Hesse, 1965) was introduced to English-speaking readers by Colin Wilson in his pretentious book *The Outsider* (1956), a text which was (deservedly) the Zeitgeist for all of ten minutes. For Wilson, 'the outsider's' purpose – be he (yes, he) saint, scholar or agitator was to remind the tedious middle classes of their moribund destiny. To that end, Harry Haller proved a telling choice for

Wilson to write about. For one thing he was foreign, continental, and so, at the time, strange and unfathomable.

Initial reactions to *Steppenwolf* were hostile. Critics pounced on its lack of structure (for instance, the absence of chapters) as well as its complexities of introversion and unreality. Here was a text operating at impenetrable levels of consciousness, its characters only loosely delineated, their interactions seemingly realistic but ultimately magical, thematic and suggestive of other (unworldly) things. That said, magic only works where there is plausibility, thus the delightfulness of its deceits. So, in *Steppenwolf,* a would-be realism takes hold but it's a realism that supports Hesse's desire to expose the unconscious life both of his characters and himself. At the same time, it is the novel's dualism, Harry as wolf and man, that makes it work so effectively at different levels. First, as an evocation of unconscious angst but, second, at a level of believability wherein Hesse threads his narrative through three (interrelated) sections. A Preface (written by a young commentator) which introduces Harry as well as providing information about the conflict that absorbs him, namely the aforementioned disgust at middle-class values plus his inability to forego the creature comforts such values bring. However, this Preface lacks adequate understanding and it is only in Part Two – when Harry recasts the preface from his own perspective – that we become privy to his psychological misgivings and the duality of his being.

When Harry, out walking, encounters a stranger, we reach the novel's third section – a 'Treatise on the Steppenwolf' – which the stranger hands to him. Whilst the Preface had yielded some essentials about Harry, and Part Two his own reflections, the Treatise transcends these by proposing a cosmic sphere – the Immortals – apprehensions of which (sphere), by Harry, calms the tensions that beset him, especially his 'bourgeois' hang-ups. For whilst Harry is plagued by opposites and the irreconcilability of his feelings and attitudes: 'The Immortals … accept chaos as the natural state of existence, for they inhabit a realm where all polarity has ceased and where every manifestation of life is approved as necessary and good' (Ziolkowski, 1977: 94).

Though this comes at the end of the novel, it pays to know that Harry will eventually obtain emotional relief, that he will be liberated from banal materialism and conformity. For now, the fate of the Steppenwolf is to be cut off from polarity. Neither to the realm of the spirits (however psychologically internalised) nor the conformity of the middle classes can he belong, and so Harry, believing himself to *be* a Steppenwolf, roams about the novel despairingly, searching for contentment but wary of how this might happen. In the end, he finds it when he stumbles into humour, when he accepts instruction on how to laugh from Hermine, an androgynous prostitute. Her message to him, that he needs her if he's going to learn to dance, to realise humour and live, is the *beginning* of a changed identity and, at the end, when she dies, his suicidalism, his commitment to despair begins to evaporate. She has infected him with life.

Another reaction to *Steppenwolf* was to see it as peculiarly German and not transferable to other cultures. But Hesse would win the Nobel Prize for literature in 1946 and by the late 50s and 60s *Steppenwolf* took off spectacularly, particularly with American students. Harry's rejection of technology and conventionality, his soul searching and distrust, mirrored the angst of 1960s youth. These, after all, were days of thunder, Woodstock, Vietnam, R.D. Laing and Timothy Leary's injunction: 'turn on, tune in, drop out', *the* mantra of the age. But *Steppenwolf* too played no mean part in fuelling the dissident's addiction to 'outsider' status. But this had its problems:

> Of all my books *Steppenwolf* is the one that was more often and more violently misunderstood than any other, and frequently it is actually the affirmative and enthusiastic readers, rather than those who rejected the book, who have reacted to it oddly.
> (Hesse, 1965: 5)

This is what happens when a book goes cult, it preys (reciprocally) on the young – some of them – reaching the parts conventional texts cannot reach, parts that despise order, celebrate nihilism whilst sniggering at optimists. Hesse said that people should take from his novel what they wanted, but he was adamant that *Steppenwolf* wasn't only about pessimism, death and destruction, that it also proffered healing, solace, redemption. Nevertheless, despite Harry's reservations, it remains *the* outsider's text expressing:

> more forcefully than any other novel by Hesse the struggle not only for self-knowledge but also for expansion outward from the discovered self. How can one come to terms with both [one's] self and with a life outside which tends to alienate, and crush the individual?
> (Norton, 1973: 53)

True, but Hesse's book was also about *becoming*, and many readers missed this, not realising that, for Hesse, as for philosophers since Plato, reaching for a balance between individual and society was worthwhile however unattainable it might be.

Choosing Steppenwolf for this book

I chose *Steppenwolf* because of the unconscious lives of its characters. Written when psychoanalysis impregnated much intellectual life, Hesse wanted to write his story in symbols. It's true that psychologists had (occasionally) attempted to write fiction (Skinner, 1976; Hudson, 1978; Yalom, 2005) but this is best left to those for whom literature is a first calling. Yet whilst Harry's predicament is a benchmark for any discussion on the asymmetry of human character, I want to lead into it, focusing on psychiatry's understanding of 'the self' in respect of duality, fragility, the tendency to split, disintegrate.

Historically, schizophrenia has been the diagnostic totem around which psychiatric theories, classical or folk, have twisted; the condition wherein 'sufferers' are designated persona non grata, their thinking demeaned by a clinical discourse that (a priori) defines it as illness. Very occasionally this has elicited dissention as when, famously, R.D. Laing (1960) reconfigured schizophrenia as 'another way of being human', not qualitatively different to anyone else. In Laing's view, so-called delusions were essential to the survival (of persons) threatened by social and professional judgements.

In the *Steppenwolf* preface, the commentator says of Harry that his: 'sickness of the soul, as I now know, is not the eccentricity of a single individual, but the sickness of the times themselves …' (Hesse, 1965: 27). This would become the (received) wisdom fuelling a secularised, radical, psychiatric, priesthood (with Laing as Archbishop) and whose starting point was that families induce madness in their young. My point is not to assert the truth of this claim but to isolate *Steppenwolf* as precursor to 1960s radical psychiatry, to show that Harry Haller personified a psychosis whose genesis was the partitioning of self from the *etiquette* of society whilst simultaneously struggling to assuage its conventions. Each chapter in this (my) book reflects more or less this historical tension between alienation and the status quo.

In the case of *Steppenwolf*, orthodox psychiatry's relegation of human stress to bio-physics and genetic funk is set against Hesse's use of Jungian analytical psychology, a powerful brand of psychiatry when he wrote his book. The contrast is the essentialist view of physical determinism versus the philosophically more challenging but productive notion of dualism, that we are possessed of both brain and mind. I want to continue assessing psychiatry's take on duality before turning to Harry Haller himself. So let's do that.

Psychiatry's dramatic personae

One such exploration begun in the 1950s concerned Multiple Personality Disorder (nowadays called Dissociative Identity Disorder) a 'condition' made up of qualitative and (incremental) quantitative elements. The qualitative aspects are the more plausible in that personality does have its multiple facets – so why not name them? – and, in any event, how often do you hear yourself exclaim, 'I'm beside myself with anger!' or, following some *faux pas,* 'That wasn't at all like me!' and so forth?

The quantitative aspect, however, *is* implausible in that its first publicised example – *Three Faces of Eve* – was about someone with three personalities (Thigpen & Cleckley, 1957) a number that has increased with each successive (celebrated) case. So that hot on the heels of *Eve* came *Sybil* (Schreiber, 1973) a woman (the disorder bypasses men) with sixteen personalities. Yet whilst the escalating mathematics proceeded apace, it was *Sybil* that eventually provoked scepticism. In 1997, Dr Herbert Spiegel, Sybil's 'backup therapist', stated that Dr Cornelia Wilbur, her principal therapist, had artificially contrived her 'personalities', that she had attached names to contrasting emotional states which Sybil dutifully acted out, shades here of *Richard III* (this volume, Chapter 5), a theatrical role played by an actor but with the part itself that of a supreme actor, illusion wrapped inside interpretation. In Sybil's case, the script was also performed by an actor/patient but with the lines scripted by a second, over-arching, performer, Dr Wilbur. Despite this, the issue (with Sybil) was less about malpractice or deception as much a naïveté endemic to psychotherapy, in this instance (apologies to Pirandello) the psychotherapist in search of many characters. As time passed, the naïveté grew and cases increased into the thousands, the number of personalities, in each successive case, shooting into the hundreds.

Pluck from the memory a rooted sorrow

Multiple Personality Disorder had come to depend for its identification on so-called 'Recovered Memory Therapy' where the aetiological significance of childhood (usually sexual) abuse was designated to be central. In fact, a therapeutic zeal fought to establish evidences of abuses even when resolutely not recalled by clients. Next, astonishing revelations, contingent on these 'evidences', began to sprout (especially in America). Grotesque abuses, sometimes spilling into communities, manifested themselves and with spiralling suspicions of satanic cults and such like. Another development, close to our purpose here, was that some of the victims of Multiple Personality Disorder reported one or more of their 'selves' taking the form of an animal. This hardly surprises since in many cultures there has prevailed a fascination with human/animal transformation myths. We have watched and read – transfixed – as the wolf becomes a grandmother, as Jekyll becomes Hyde or as a Full Moon brings the wolf out in others. The advent of science and technology induced fascination with the potentially negative uses to which these might be put. Eccentric scientists began to crop up in novels, usually hellbent on creating monsters, destroying vampires or, more recently, constructing malevolent humanoid robots (Proyas, 2004).

No doubt the Darwinian theory of evolution played a part in this as today are there fears that genetic research may incur horrific outcomes and mutations. Many issues arise here, but perhaps the most salient (for the layperson at least) is injunction. Do not wander off the beaten track, don't go into the woods, don't meddle with nature, cherish what is natural, unsullied, beware what changes form. We will discuss further the monstrous/wolverine as human but, as a preliminary exercise:

Doppelgänger syndrome

An unusual phenomenon, though well established in the psychiatric literature (Enoch & Ball, 2001), Doppelgängers believe they are being replaced by someone else, that their mirror image is in a process of becoming. The belief begins in noticing similarities between themselves and a 'stranger' but with a growing realisation that 'strangers are us'. Its creepiness is creepiest in Dostoevsky's *The Double* (1972) where Mr Golyadkin, walking home one night, thinks he sees someone he knows. The someone becomes increasingly recognisable and so naturally Mr Golyadkin follows him until, astonishingly, they both end up in Mr Golyadkin's house where:

> Everything he had feared and foreseen had now become cold reality. It took his breath away and made his head whirl. The unknown, also still in hat and overcoat, was sitting before him on his own bed, and with a slight smile on his lips; narrowing his eyes a little, he gave him a friendly nod. Mr Golyadkin wanted to cry out, but could not, to make some sort of protest but his strength failed him. His hair stood on end and he collapsed on to a chair, insensible with horror. Mr Golyadkin had recognised his nocturnal acquaintance. Mr Golyadkin's nocturnal acquaintance was none other than himself, Mr Golyadkin himself, another Mr Golyadkin, but exactly the same as himself – in short, in every respect what is called his double …
> (pp. 172–3)

This descent into madness is persuasive because of the step-by-step access to Mr Golyadkin's feelings and suspicions it provides. You might compare Dostoevsky's method to Gilman's in *The Yellow Wallpaper* (this volume, Chapter 6), another 'insider' testimony to encroaching insanity and where the heroine, out walking, 'sees' people or where, ensconced in bed, her wallpaper becomes animate, encroaching, threatening.

Whilst psychiatry categorised these experiences as mental illnesses, ignoring the beliefs of those involved, close encounters and transformations stalk the novels of Hesse and Dostoevsky as they have literature since the ancients (see Kyziridis, 2005). Psychiatric theory defines these matters as delusions and hallucinations and it does so to ensure the application of its physical cures and therapies. It's time to see how we can add to this and so we must now turn to:

Steppenwolf and the strange case of Harry Haller

We don't know where Harry comes from. There are hints in the Preface, but they tell us zilch about his background, his history. *Steppenwolf* was published in Germany in 1927 but you wouldn't think so given the paucity of contextual information in it, whether political, economic, or social. For example, there is no mention of the recent slaughter of World War One, you don't get the sense of imminent economic collapse in Europe or the impending rise of Nazism. Rather is it a fiction which dwells on individual psychology and the desire to reconcile tensions between artistic expression and social order. Hesse sustains this centuries-old tension by recourse to Jungian types and mythologies but which in human terms takes its starting point from personal consciousness.

A Protestant ethic

Whereas, before, political states took account of religious imperatives, man now genuflects before a moral order that takes account of relativism. In the twentieth century, relativism would resource the development of psychotherapy, to the extent that a new cluster of philosophers – 'experts in human nature' – took centre stage. Condemning expertise, these 'experts' constructed a psychotherapy which they called humanistic. It is with Carl Ransom Rogers (1951) and 'person-centredness' that the relationship between the individual and society is redefined from political to psychological terms and in a disarmingly attractive way. Universally revered by today's 'helping professions', the darker implications of Rogerianism were concurrently shunned. For example, its Protestant, Calvinist, ethic of accounting one's consciousness before God – Luther's declaration: 'Here I stand, I can do no other' (or: is it, I *will* do no other?) – is a truer basis for what drives it, an unashamed commitment to putting private (emotional) ambitions ahead of everything else.

In more ways than one Rogers recasts the Nietzschean dream as a harmless means of achieving 'self-actualisation'. All three: Nietzsche, Hesse, and Rogers were closely conjoined with Protestantism. Both Rogers and Nietzsche attended theological college and Hesse's father and grandfather were religious ministers as was Nietzsche's father. Whilst they carried religious baggage in different ways, an essential commitment to individualism drove their propositions and conclusions. Nietzsche rejected the religion of his fathers. Declining the old morality he pronounced God dead, imploring man to enter history on his own terms. The old religions, argued Nietzsche, had stopped human progress in its tracks, especially Christianity with its penchant for helping the weak instead of (more profitably) celebrating the strong. Although Nietzsche's Superman (Übermensch) was realised most horrifically, in our own time, by the Nazis, the impulse to stomp on others continues. We have reflected on the murderous, if guilt-laden, power scrambles of General Macbeth (this volume, Chapter 9) and more so with the sinisterly comic-genius King Richard (this volume, Chapter 5): indeed, as Bryan Magee (1998: 178) notes: all of Shakespeare (and so all of life) flows from a few lines in *Richard III*:

> Conscience is but a word that cowards use. Devised at first to keep the strong in awe. Our strong arms be our conscience, swords our law!

Rogerian psychology denies this, pushing instead a false consciousness, a banal soliloquy on human goodness, a predilection for optimism, a utopianism of individuals. So, in twentieth-century psychology, did Rogers combine a cynical diligence (worthy of Richard) with a convivial regard (the 'person') albeit with scant notice of the mores of the wider society. Nonetheless, his influence was enormous, virtually establishing 'counselling' as an independent form of human enquiry.

Although – in *Steppenwolf* (1965) – Hesse cuts his readers off from particular times and cultures, his alter ego, Harry, quests for a meaning to his particular existence. Embracing the Nietzschian affirmation that suffering one's way through, facing one's troubles stoically is what matters, he struggles through them for the sake of it, declaring that: 'a man should be proud of suffering. All suffering is a reminder of our high estate' (p. 21) or an expression of a need to suffer, to *be* suffering as an emotional guarantee of some sort of meaningful life. As the first narrator says (p. 15) of him: 'Haller was a genius of suffering, and that in the meaning of many sayings of Nietzsche, he had created within himself an ingenious, a boundless and frightful capacity for pain.'

And so:

Disconsolate, tramping the streets, morose, fearing death, desiring death, Harry meets a stranger who hands him a 'Treatise on the Steppenwolf'. Imagine that! Can you believe that? Here is a middle-aged man, living a problematic middle-class life, somewhere in Germany, an academic, human, not beast, yet beastly, a Steppenwolf who thinks he's blessed because compelled to pursue knowledge through to perfection. And now, a stranger hands him a dissertation on his own nature, a treatise which, if true, could only have been written by himself. So why has he been handed this by a stranger? Is it simply to further a novel of which the treatise is now a part?

Or, *has* he met a stranger? The stranger has appeared from nowhere, faceless, saying little, just as quickly disappearing. It's an odd encounter and hugely improbable in real terms. Note, as well, that the stranger doesn't offer the treatise: rather does Harry request something from inside the stranger's box. What was he hoping to get? What did he imagine was inside this box?

Until now, the sustaining motif of the novel has been Harry's disdain for middle-class ordure, for homes that: 'smell of turpentine and soap and where there is panic if you bang the door or come in with dirty shoes' (p. 36). That said, his 'sentimental weakness' for 'quiet and order, cleanliness and respectable domesticity' (p. 36) can't prize him from society's coffee bars, its American cinema and its theatres, and he surmises (p. 39) that if people actually like these, then: 'I am wrong, I am crazy. I am in truth the Steppenwolf that I often call myself, the beast astray who finds neither home nor joy nor nourishment in a world that is strange and incomprehensible.' In fact, there is much about Harry that is inexplicable. Jazz music, for instance – 'hot and raw as the steam of raw flesh' (p. 46) – he loathes, yet it exerts its 'secret charms' on him. Like himself, jazz music is two-fold, its duality claiming him sensually but repulsing him intellectually. This is music from another world and another race, new, fresh, sweeping away older, different, European antecedents (see the conversation between Harry and Pablo pp. 155–7).

Perforce, in this novel, everything is at 'sixes and sevens', persons, cultures, genders, histories, continents, religions. But it is the handing over of the treatise that constitutes the final break with reality for, from here on in, matters become even more complex, dreamy and unpredictable. The treatise informs Harry that a human/Steppenwolf duality is simplistic, that man is comprised of 'a thousand selves' and ultimately accountable to none in particular. Such talk risks dissembling into metaphysics and impenetrableness. What prevents this is the hook with psychology, specifically the connection with Jung's (1968) 'collective unconscious', its signs, symbols and timelessness.

Some notes on psychiatry and Hesse

So: when reading *Steppenwolf*, a working knowledge of Jungian psychology, especially the 'collective unconscious', will help. Many of Hesse's ideas are best understood through this concept, particularly the contention that psychological dispositions reflect universal *archetypes,* symbolic images reflected in religions, dreams, art, mythology, and which determine the developmental stages of the life span. One of these, the *shadow*, acts as a repressed metaphor at odds with – but not entirely cut off from – conscious awareness. You will encounter this *shadow* in your dreams for example, where it constantly grapples towards a resolution of your everyday concerns in symbolic terms. Instinctive, irrational, the Jungian unconscious apprehends its environment via a hypersensitivity to smells, temperatures, sights and sounds, in fact the whole of physicality and emotion. It was this which led Hesse to write *Steppenwolf*, to make meaningful, in human terms, the primitive recognition that the inexplicable reconciles the obnoxious with the desirable, thus bringing about the unpalatable pronouncements of those called schizophrenic.

Ancestral images

Jung (1968) was dogged by ancestral imagery and his referencing of it has not stood him in good stead. For instance, he says of the *shadow* that it is dark-featured and this opens doors to sinister interpretation. At this point, a warning: historical scholarship has identified Jung as a Nazi sympathiser. That being the case, his views on 'dark-skinned' ancestral races – the notion that 'dark' implies inferiority or negativity – means that his general 'psychology' be approached with care.

This mattered less when Hesse wrote his book. But even had it done, it's difficult to imagine a *Steppenwolf* which disavows Jungian philosophy altogether. Shorn of its racial underpinnings, there would still be enough left to push the novel along such as, for instance, Hesse's use of the Anima, the feminine 'side' of the male. Whilst the animus is that which males present to the world, a feminine impulse must needs find expression in male psychology too. In this context, pay attention to the female characters in *Steppenwolf* and try to work out points of connection between them and Harry. Watch Hesse manoeuvre his characters inside the 'story line'. To what extent, and in what sense, are they separate people? Occasionally some of the characters display such uncanny insight into Harry's thinking, you might well believe that he's talking to himself. For example, look how Hermine reads Harry's mind. She can make him guess her name correctly and though different to him, as chalk is to cheese, she knows him intimately. She is inside him. At the same time, other aspects of the novel's characters, including Hermine's, not only support its Jungian undertow but, as well: 'demonstrate qualities of humanness [by leading Harry] away from his self-destructive urges towards a new understanding of life' (Norton, 1973: 55).

Infatuation

Hesse's infatuation with Jungian psychology wasn't idiosyncratic or self-serving – he had had analytic sessions with Dr. J.B. Lang, a pupil of Jung, and he was of an age, when writing his novel, when Jungian therapy is at its most therapeutic, the middle years. As Maier (1953: 10) noted:

> Approaching forty years of age, in the midst of the First World War, Hesse lived in total isolation, unable to cope with the impasse he had reached. His surroundings had lost all importance for him: that is, in terms of Jungian psychology, libido had been withdrawn from the outside world and, turning inward, was endowing with energy the archetypes which, in turn, threatened to overwhelm him and hold him in darkness.

Realising that the archetypes, their destructiveness, were rooted in humankind generally allowed Hesse to recognise, through therapy, a need to re-align himself more conscientiously with others. These autobiographical elements back Hesse's claim that *Steppenwolf* is a work of optimism, not despair.

Literary influences

In some respects it doesn't have any. Although its intense preoccupation with human motivation was rare in novels up till then, it is not unique in its use of multiple perspectives or layered textuality. At a stretch, one sees these elements germinate in works like *Frankenstein* (Shelley, 2006) or *Jekyll and Hyde*

139

(Stevenson, 1979), human transformation novels that reflected progressions in neurology during the nineteenth century, particularly investigations of the brain. According to Harrington (1987:17), at this time physicians were starting to ask:

> Whether ... circumstances might arise in which each [brain] hemisphere could take on an independent life of its own. It seemed particularly plausible to suppose that one brain-half might fall prey to a delusion whilst the other remained healthy.

That madness might inhabit specific brain areas intrigued Franz Joseph Gall (1758–1828), founder of phrenology, who began treating problems that were, he claimed, located respectively in the left and right sides of the brain. At the time, it wasn't uncommon for people to view things as polar opposites – religion versus Darwinism, for example – or authority versus freedom and so on. Harrington (1987) notes that Masao Miyoshi (1969: 106–7) develops:

> this thesis through analysis of such literary conceits and themes as the Doppelgänger, the double, the polarisation of evil and wholesomeness within the gothic villain/hero, the romantic 'other self', the Jekyll and Hyde split personality, the identity crisis of the self-alienated hero.

In fact, what prevented neurologists advocating a complete anatomical scheme (of life) was the still persuasive hold of 'the spiritual' over human thought. But, more so, did experimentation promote conflictive ideas of localisation, separateness and even duplicity within human brains and this contradicted the unity of man inhabiting a soul. Yet experimentation fascinated people and they lapped up its imagined, fantastic, consequences. For example, inducing unusual behaviours via hypnosis was causing a sensation in Paris and public demonstrations of people forgetting things they had just said and done also belittled the idea of a brain at one with itself. Some of these discoveries were so fundamental as to be understood by fiction writers who quickly saw their potential within story lines.

In a sense, what Robert Louis Stevenson does, in *Jekyll and Hyde*, is write a neurological version of Hesse's psychoanalytic journey, the latter at the mercy of metaphor, mythology and the psyche, the former impelled by chemistry and emergent knowledge of brain structure. These two dimensions, brilliantly evoked by Sebastian Faulkes' (2006) novel *Human Traces*, mirrored the duality within the development of psychiatric theory reflecting the dichotomy between the biological and the psychological. What they held in common, in a post-Enlightenment world, was a serious challenge to the religious view of life. Why be surprised if nineteenth-century readers feared losing a common morality grounded in salvation. The new thinking, be it mental archetypes or brain tissue, left little room for the soul and even if, in *Steppenwolf*, Harry turns to 'the

Immortals' these too – the Mozarts and Goethes – are of this world, their status emerging from human action, art transforming life.

Conclusion

Theme one: Psychology

Ambivalence in *Steppenwolf* is Hesse's way of establishing identity in fiction. Characters like Hermine, Pablo and Maria are suppressions of Harry Haller's unconscious. Their sensuous and intellectual encounters with him, realised in narrative form, are what bring him to a new way of living:

> The way to innocence, and to the 'yet to be created', and to God, does not
> lean backwards, but forwards, not to the wolf or to the child, but ever further
> into responsibility, ever deeper into the process of becoming a human being.
>   (Hesse, 1965: 249)

Hesse had learned this from therapy. Jung, in turn, saw Hesse's novel as espousing the spirit of his version of psychoanalysis. For example, on entering the Magic Theatre – 'entering psychoanalysis' – Hesse/Haller is exposed, via the mirrors, to a hundred splintered illuminations of *their* psyches. Rather than relate this realistically, Hesse communicates it iconically by fictional incongruence and improbability. His female 'characters' may be, at once, feminine alter egos (or anima), but they possess sufficient characterological strength in traditional story terms to carry the (story and) reader along. Not perhaps as easy a read as my other choices, and there were times when I found the timelessness and the idiosyncrasies wearying. But worth sticking with and, when finished, not an easy book to get out of your head.

Theme two: The artist

A central question of this (my) book is the relationship between an author and his/her book and few explicate this more than *Steppenwolf,* where Harry Haller (Herman Hesse) wrestles with multiple spiritual, psychological, social and artistic metaphors of social unpleasantness. The relationship between life and art has engendered questions of nature's reality and interpretation since criticism began. Hesse deals with this by moving literary goalposts, blurring connections between the inner and relational worlds of his characters, especially Harry. This leaves the reader perplexed at times but it lies at the heart of why insoluble dilemmas beset human choices.

Coda

Steppenwolf is about the bond between artist and art and, in the run-up to writing it, Hesse had come to see himself as a 'Protestant Steppenwolf', which is to say that writing fiction allowed him to transform and make manifest his neurosis. So his inability to recover from marriage breakdown and physical illness is distilled in a narrative of hope and anticipation. R.D. Laing (1960: 44) captures this in his take on the ontological anxiety of schizophrenia:

> If the individual cannot take the realities, aliveness, autonomy, and identity of himself and others for granted, then he has to become absorbed in contriving ways of trying to be real, of keeping himself or others alive, of preserving his identity, in efforts, as he will often put it, to prevent himself losing himself.

Hesse finds himself in his fiction. His is no dry account of a breakdown which might or might not add to theories about alienation. It is an art work, a skeleton (realist) novel that explores aesthetic and psychological incongruence in unconscious humanity. It teaches our senses.

Films

A film version of *Steppenwolf* was released in 1974 directed by Fred Haines and starring Max von Sydow as Harry and Dominique Sanda as Hermine. Hesse part wrote the script (with Haines) and critics thought that the film fairly reflected the themes of the novel. The main problem, of course, was how to communicate Harry's brooding philosophising but this was mostly resolved through von Sydow's outstanding performance.

Three Faces of Eve was directed by Nunnally Johnsone and released in 1957 starring Joanne Woodward as Eve, a role for which she won both Academy and Golden Globe Awards. It was this movie which popularised Multiple Personality Disorder as both feasible and not uncommon. The film was based on the novel of the same name by psychiatrists Corbet Hilsman Thigpen and Hervey Milton Cleckley who also wrote the movie's script.

Sybil, directed by Daniel Petrie, was released as a Television movie in 1974. The protagonist was played by Sally Field with, intriguingly, her psychiatrist, Doctor Wilbur, played by none other than Joanne Woodward who had earlier played Eve. Again, the film did much to solidify Multiple Personality Disorder as a psychotic syndrome, predominantly a disorder of females and inescapably linked to childhood sexual abuse by men.

Dr Jekyll and Mr Hyde, directed by Reuben Mamoulian and starring Frederic March, remains the definitive film of Stevenson's story. The simian appearance of Hyde has greatly influenced our visual perspective of the story. It was an image intended to convey the repression of evil, not surprisingly given that the

1930s was the heyday of psychoanalysis, including its influence on film makers. The transformation from Jekyll to Hyde is truly astonishing (for its time) and it was years before the cinematic methods used to achieve it were made known.

Unlike previous interpretations, Mamoulian's film addresses the sexual undertones of the story, especially the idea that to inhibit desire because of social mores will induce transformative evil. Like Richard III: 'And therefore, since I cannot prove a lover I am determined to prove a villain', Hyde, far from being liberated through repression, turns monstrous. Whereas Jekyll relates (erotically) to women, Hyde seeks to savage them. Material removed for the 1930s release has been restored to the VHS and DVD versions.

I, Robot, directed by Alex Proyas, released in 2004, was a big hit. It followed the Frankenstein premise of creating something, in this case a robot, with the intention of benefiting mankind but only for the robot to self-discover that he/she might be better off fending for itself. It's the standard conundrum of humanoid technology; will the computerised robot reach a point of intelligence wherein it declares independence unilaterally?

References

Brown, GW & Harris, T (1978) *The Social Origins of Depression*. London: Tavistock.

Dostoevsky, F (1972) *Notes from the Underground [and] The Double*. London: Penguin Modern Classics.

Durkheim, E (1989) *Suicide: A study in sociology*. London: Routledge.

Enoch, D & Ball, H (2001) *Uncommon Psychiatric Syndromes*. London: Arnold.

Faulkes, S (2006) Human Trace. London: Vintage.

Haines, F (1974) *Steppenwolf* [film]. Peter Spragus Films.

Harrington, A (1987) *Medicine, Mind, and the Double Brain*. Princeton, NJ: Princeton University Press.

Hesse, H (1965) *Steppenwolf*. Harmondsworth: Penguin. [Original work published 1927]

Hudson, L (1978) *The Nympholepts*. London: Cape.

Johnsone, N (1957) *The Three Faces of Eve* [film]. Hollywood: Twentieth-Century Fox.

Jung, CG (1968) *The Archetypes and the Collective Unconscious*. London: Routledge.

Kipling, R (2007) *The Second Jungle Book*. Charleston, SC: Biblio Bazaar.

Kyziridis, TC (2005) Notes on the history of schizophrenia. *German Journal of Psychiatry, 8* (3), 42–8.

Laing, RD (1960) *The Divided Self*. London: Tavistock Publications.

Magee, B (1998) *The Story of Philosophy*. London: Dorling Kindersley.

Maier, E (1953) *The Psychology of CG Jung and the Works of Hermann Hesse*. Unpublished Thesis submitted in fulfilment of Doctor of Philosophy Degree to Graduate School of Arts and Sciences. New York: New York University. Available online at: www.gas.ucsb.edu/projects/hesse/papers/maier.pdf

Mamoulian, R (1931) *Dr Jekyll and Mr Hyde*. Hollywood: Paramount Pictures.

Miyoshi, M (1969) *The Divided Self: A perspective on the literature of the Victorians*. New York: New York University Press.

Norton, RC (1973) *Hermann Hesse's Futuristic Idealism*. Bern: Herbert Lang & Co.

Petrie, D (1976) *Sybil* [film]. USA: NBC Television.

Proyas, A (2004) *I, Robot* [film]. Hollywood: Canlaws Productions.

Rogers, CR (1951) *Client-Centred Therapy*. London: Constable.

Schreiber, FR (1973) *Sybil*. London: Allen Lane.

Shelley, M (2006) *Frankenstein*. London: Bloomsbury Classics.

Skinner, BF (1976) *Walden Two*. London: Macmillan.

Stevenson, RL (1979) *The Strange Case of Dr Jekyll and Mr Hyde*. London: Penguin Classics.

Thigpen, CH & Cleckley, HM (1957) *The Three Faces of Eve*. London: Secker & Warburg.

Wilson, C (1956) *The Outsider*. London: Gollancz.

Yalom, I (2005) *The Schopenhauer Cure*. New York: HarperCollins.

Ziolkowski, T (1977) Herman Hesse's Steppenwolf: A sonata in prose. In J Liebmann (ed), *Hermann Hesse: A collection of criticism* (pp 90–109). New York: McGraw-Hill.

CHAPTER 11

ASYLUM

The wicked lie in wait for the righteous; seeking their very lives.
  (*Psalms,* 37: 32)

Stark, staring mad.
  (John Dryden, 1812, *The Satires of Persius Flaccus*)

Synopsis

Stella Raphael arrives at a 1950s forensic psychiatric hospital, the wife of Max, its newly appointed deputy superintendent who is glad of the move because it is good for his career. Stella is more reluctant but, for now, is a dutiful wife and mother to their young son, Charlie. Wanting to spruce up the surroundings of their hospital house, Max arranges for Edgar Stark, a patient of fellow psychiatrist Peter Cleave, to work on an outhouse. Stark murdered his wife by beheading her and then gouging out her eyes.

   Stella falls heels over head for Stark and they begin an affair. It is one of the (minor) uncertainties of the novel that Stella and Edgar have sex here there and everywhere on the hospital grounds, even in Max and Stella's bedroom, without anyone noticing. For those of you who worked in the big asylum/ hospitals, as I did, you may find this far-fetched. On the other hand, the stupendousness of their behaviour may have so beggared belief that it passed unnoticed. Oh: on his 'visit' to Stella's bedroom Stark steals Max's clothes and escapes to London.

   Despite knowing his past, Stella follows him and they shack up in squalid surroundings owned by one of his friends. After a time, frightened that he may kill her, she steals away but returns after a few days only to be met by the police. Returned to the hospital, she appears to sink into a kind of depression. Loathing Max, they nevertheless settle into a tense liaison possibly for Charlie's sake. Following suspicion that Max had delayed reporting Edgar's escape he is dismissed from his job and decides to move to a hospital in Wales. Following the move Stella continues in a kind of doldrums and allows herself to have sex with a neighbour because he simply asks for it.

   On a school outing to the local moors, Charlie gets into trouble in a pond as Stella stands by watching him drown. She is taken to the hospital where the affair with Stark began, this time as a patient of Peter Cleave who tells her

145

that Stark is not in the hospital, though he is. Cleave attempts to treat her but also offers his hand in marriage which she accepts. As part of her rehabilitation she attends the annual hospital dance wearing the same dark dress she wore when, the year before, she danced with Stark allowing him to press his erection against her. That night she swallows sufficient (hoarded) tablets, dies and is buried in the hospital grounds. Now let's add in some background to these events.

Background

Something that's always struck me about male psychiatrists is that compared to other medical specialists they take first prize for smugness. They exude a self-assurance hardly comparable to the contentious act of defining some human behaviours as illness so as to (frequently) treat these via legal detention and coercion. In addition, psychiatry operates from a knowledge base that is as rudimentary as it is fragmented and betimes misplaced. Further, there is the eagerness of some of its representatives to impress us with an understanding of all things human. Think Raj Persaud, ensconced on the 'good morning' TV sofa, pontificating on any and all human foibles. Or the late Anthony Clare who, having called Freud a 'confidence trickster', nevertheless donned the mantle of psychological inquisitor to the rich and famous in BBC Radio Four's *In the Psychiatrist's Chair*. It wasn't much of an inquisition really, more a series of comfortable chats but with the added gravitas of a would-be nineteenth century Viennese consulting room.

The gravitas came largely from popular media, especially films and television. I remember well the 1963–1964 television series *The Human Jungle*, starring Herbert Lom as the charismatic psychiatrist Dr Corder – so charismatic in fact that hundreds of letters arrived on the *actor's* desk every week requesting help! The programme was remarkable for an opening sequence that heralded profundity and erudition, Corder sitting behind an enormous mahogany desk swathed in cigarette smoke and dead-pan seriousness, notions of 'the psychiatrist' descended from Mount Olympus, pontificates on the human condition at the ready. McGrath casts his narrator Dr Peter Cleave in the same mould: 'I wanted the reader to come to trust Cleave, so that he was believable as a compassionate, wise, sort of detached psychiatrist. Everything a psychiatrist is supposed to be' (Lowman, 1997). Supposed to be? On page 24 McGrath's comment about psychiatrists suggests a favourable view of their powers, to put it mildly. It happens when Stella, having just had sex with Stark, encounters Max. Forced into over-familiarity because intuiting his sense that something is wrong she realises that any openness between them must, from here on, be guarded against: 'And that her explosive secret must be hidden with especial skill from the eyes of this sudden stranger with his *desperately acute powers of mental intrusion and perception*' [my italics].

And again (p. 154) note Stella's observation that any average psychiatrist could diagnose heartbreak with ease. Actually, I am unsure that heartbreak has ever featured on any curriculum for budding psychiatrists. I suspect that McGrath has been unduly influenced by his father, reputedly a wise and discerning (certainly liberal) psychiatrist. Having said that, in order to make the symbolic elements of the narrative work, he must/needs imbue his main medical character with insight, at least where others are concerned.

Given the therapy that Cleave wishes to do with Edgar plus his declaration of professional interest in the novel's opening sentence, we can suppose him a student of Freud. Undoubtedly, his narration of the novel's characters and events is intended as the voice of reason, of psychiatry, effecting the condescending detachment common to the trade. It becomes apparent however the he is not to be trusted, that there is more to his account of things than meets the eye. The 'unreliable narrator' is an established (literary) ruse (see this volume, Chapters 1 and 13) intended to lull the reader into a sense of security. With Cleave, we slowly apprehend that behind supposed wisdom lies little more than rudimentary clinical maxims.

This is hardly surprising given how psychiatrists are prepared for their role. Having studied physics, chemistry and/or biology at secondary school they move on to university for five years of medical training. On acquiring a medical licence, *less than one per cent* opt to specialise in psychiatry, a factor of philosophical as well as economic importance, though rarely addressed (by the psychiatric profession) as such. There then follows another three years of preparation for membership of the Royal College of Psychiatrists but which requires not a whit of training in interpersonal relationships, little of self-reflection, or what it means to be human. Such diversions might inhibit the self-assuredness provided by membership of a medical model of madness. Alternatively, of course, the hyped confidence may simply compensate for psychiatrists' self-perceived fragility compared with the knowledge base and status of other medical specialities. Lastly, in terms of the long-lasting fear of, and stigma attached to, the insane, it's not surprising that those responsible for their containment should be accorded power and authority by the wider society. This is a façade which has only now begun to show some cracks and points of departure. But, for years, and especially in the era of the mental hospitals, the kingship of the (mostly) male doctors was unchallengeable. This bears heavily on what follows, the tale of Stella Raphael, a psychiatrist's wife, and her sexual dalliance with Edgar Stark, a hospitalised, violent, patient.

Beginnings

Patrick McGrath was born in 1950, the son of the Medical Superintendent of Broadmoor Hospital, a maximum security psychiatric unit. Growing up within the hospital grounds he was in daily contact with Broadmoor's inmates. Yet he claims: 'There is nothing I ever remember as a manifestation of insanity' (Tonkin, 2000). This might be because he only encountered trustees, patients whose institutional careers had rendered them 'burnt out': that is, lacking volition, interest, unable to progress beyond repetitive, mundane, tasks. It's equally possible that McGrath had repressed what, in childhood, was uncomfortable or unfathomable to him, his novels compromising truths wherein is projected intolerable anxieties through his character's mad, bad and dangerous relationships.

Kakutani (1997) agrees that McGrath's twin preoccupations with sex and death, control and obsession, the fascination with morbidity, are unconscious speculations on his part. In this, we are in receipt of writing that starts from a repressed consciousness that has 'witnessed' madness at first hand. We, in turn, confronted with such a text, cannot but allow that *our* responses similarly harbour unpleasant motives in our wanting to read it. Unsurprisingly, McGrath's novels have been called 'gothic', elegant blends of repulsion, passion, secrecy and obsession burbling within stifling settings. Specifically, McGrath is a master of what McWilliam (2000) calls 'credible gothic' which is that his stories are believable but also disconcerting in their symbolic renditions of violence. In other words, this is no mere horror show but follows the gothic tradition of Edgar Allen Poe – Stella's lover is called Edgar – wherein madness is contained by the values, the beliefs, of the ruling class of doctors, and their attendants, a hierarchy where everyone knows their station as well as their obligation to the maintenance of sameness. The asylum becomes a metaphor for the safety that comes from social cohesion, from adherence to hospital etiquette and the wider moral order. Violate these, says the story, and the outcomes will be catastrophic.

The setting

Asylum is set in a Victorian-built hospital. As such, given McGrath's family background, it would have been difficult for him to get things wrong in the detail. So if you want an insider's account of hospital life in the 1950s, the tail end of the asylum/hospital trajectory, this is the book for you. It's beautifully written, firstly with exemplary attention to syntax and tone, and secondly, from a distance which lends it clarity and restraint. Thirdly, its different characters so second-naturedly go about their roles that one sees how the 'totalising characteristics' vividly described by Goffman (1968) could dictate everyday institutional behaviour. Hospital life was a choreography of set pieces, everyone knowing their duty, *compliant*. The golden rule, elevated to a bespoke paranoia, was separation of male and female, staff and patients, the latter by its nature a separation of species, a psychological apartheid born of a dread of emotional contact with 'the mad'. Laing (1985: 123) writes about this entertainingly:

The staff had strict orders not to talk to the patients or to encourage the patients to talk to them, or to each other, or to themselves, or at all. Talking between patients was observed, reported and broken up. You must not let a schizophrenic talk to you. It aggravates the psychotic process. As in bone fractures, so in fractured minds: immobilisation is the answer.

Younger readers may be struck by the harshness of this. For example, by Mrs Bain's disdain (p. 14) at the *idea* of a patient entering a staff space without invite. Equally, her dismay that Edgar Stark addresses Mrs Raphael by her first name. But the fact is, Stella Raphael's familiarity with the patient Stark, quite apart from any intimacy, would have been seen as truly shocking.

The nature of how, when and where patients interacted with staff was empirically examined by Annie Altschul (1972) who found that lines of demarcation between psychiatric nurses and patients were geographically distinct. Whilst staff had access to most areas of a ward or unit, patients were restricted to designated areas with the kitchen off limits except by permission. Similarly, the ward office was virgin territory for patients unless under special invite, which was rare. An interesting finding from Clarke and Flanagan's (2003) qualitative investigation of five psychiatric units in South-East England was that significantly little had changed in respect of patient-nurse interaction including the exclusivity of 'the office', albeit today's obsession with paperwork accentuates the staff's need for seclusion.

So that when, in *Asylum*, an illicit affair breaks out between a psychiatrist's wife and a patient, the tramlines of custom hit the buffers big time. The strength of fiction is to take the temperature of such events (and their effects) and convey these in creatively persuasive ways, something that nonfiction doesn't do that well. Indeed, it is remarkable how, in nonfiction history texts, the sexual lives of hospital populations are hardly mentioned. In fairness, this was, after all, the 1950s, a different world to ours in matters of moral propriety and especially sexual expression. We today are the post-Sixties children of Marx and Coca Cola, the questionable beneficiaries of a momentous change in the cultural acceptance of matters previously frowned upon. As novelist Malcolm Bradbury (1975: 24) describes things in his novel *The History Man*, something happened around the time of the Sixties. In the personages of Howard and Barbara Kirk, his novel shows how they switched from Fifties parochialism to Sixties radical chic:

What happened? Well ... the walls of limitation they had been living inside began to give way; they both started to vibrate with new desires and expectations. They laughed more, and challenged people more ... and what had done this to the Kirks? Well, to understand it you need to know a little Marx, a little Freud, and a little social history ... and the human capacity of consciousness to expand and explode

And if you happened to be a radical psychiatrist, the expansion was into consciousness, with ideological bombs hurled at the walls of psychiatric oppression. But you could count such psychiatrists on one hand and you can rest assured that Stella Raphael's husband wasn't one of them. Indeed, Max Raphael represents a counter-reformation against radical psychiatry that was already contained within it. This is in the nature of revolution, a tendency to breed dissent against the very act of revolting. Conventional psychiatric practice continued along its urbane, confident way, as it knew it would and, in this novel, perfectly embodied in Peter Cleave. There he is, ensconced on the margins of the story, passing judgements, moulding his observations, coming to conclusions. Ambiguous from the start – what's his sexuality for instance? – one never knows when or how to trust him. Note Cleave's calm exposition, the smugness of which we spoke earlier. In the face of distress, his is a distant, clinical, veneer, a fitting seer into the fate of the other characters and the outcomes of their actions. It's all on page one: the opening, preening, sentence, his definitions of *types* of behaviour, his succinct descriptions, the patronising tone, the male chauvinism, the moral injunctions. But, as we shall discover, Cleave is a schemer, he plays with people and is not to be trusted with colleagues, nor indeed with anyone. For instance, he provides (p. 37) Max's dominant mother, Brenda, with reports on her son, frequently speaking to her by phone. Playing his cards close to his chest, he airily brushes aside all queries and suggestions about his own ambition. In fact, Cleave has always wanted to run the place, no more so than now, nearing retirement. But Max stands in his way and Max has a wife.

Cleave's ambition is wrapped up in his unreliability as the novel's narrator. But, as well, he seems intrinsically unable to engage people in any depth, rather deciphering them from a distance, pleased with his analytic abilities, the power to define people as ill. He believes especially that when people deviate from civilised values, be these values a sham, they tinker with their own sanity. What some people might call love, the Cleaves of this world see as madness. Maybe they know something, what it means to be 'madly in love' for instance, or to be an 'incurable' romantic. Cleave fears romantics where all is passion, glands in full flow, no time to think, emotional disaster beckoning.

Cleave's orientation as a psychiatrist may seem unusual for someone working in one of the big asylums of the Fifties. However, psychoanalysis was a major force in English psychiatry during the 1930s when many of the asylum doctors would have been newly qualified. Clearly, Cleave has had some training in psychoanalysis: there are references to 'transference' (p. 40) where Edgar confides in Cleave as a father figure about previously repressed motives, and we are clearly meant to see displacement at play (p. 47) when Stella ruminates on how the aggressive forces of the institution take Edgar from her as though he were her child, an ominous sense of apprehension here of what may happen later. So, perhaps we need Cleave in that he provides a kind of reason, an analytic thread that carries the story forward. But he is intellectually dishonest, his actions mediated via machination and deceit.

The start of the affair

Cleave (p. 13) traces the origins of the affair to Stella's persistent failure to mention her infatuation even when impropriety has not yet occurred. He believes that keeping her feelings from Max is tantamount to betrayal. The annual dance which commences and ends the novel (and the affair) is pivotal; Stella's acceptance of Edgar's sexuality at the beginning and then her public testament to him at the end constituting the story. Note, though, as Cleave tells it, that the main deception has been against *him* and that it's not thrashing libidos that jealously offends him as much as Edgar's jeopardising their therapeutic relationship, *their* time together.

An annual ball indeed took place in most asylums. Less a loosening of 'the rules' it was more their re-emphasis, the 'freedom' of the occasion ostensible, the staff contriving false bonhomie. Any encounter between staff and patients outside the determinants of their roles were always nervous affairs. Stark's sexual advance on Stella, in the midst of staff surveillance, however camouflaged, is daring except that he has 'read' her accurately and calculated well her sexual response to him.

Throughout, Cleave sees Edgar as manipulative, not passionate, using his sexual prowess to gain control of the wife of a deputy superintendent. Resentful that Stark has forsaken his therapy, a therapy designed to strip away his defences and his self-delusions, to force him to confront what he had done, Cleave decides to monitor their sexual liaison, fascinated that it repeats that violence which Stark visited upon his wife. This is the voyeuristic undertow of psychiatry, the longing that others be 'mad for me', to act out what the onlooker has suppressed. Thus the construction of diagnostic types within which reside (in part) the projected self-loathing of a psychological confederacy ill at ease with its professional judgements.

Edgar Stark and the myth of the genius/lunatic

McGrath pulls few punches with the character Stark. Here, indisputably is a madman, the clichéd dangerous lunatic who has beheaded a wife, gouged out her eyes (all the more for having looked at him) before sitting down beside her for a chat. He killed – according to psychiatry – from delusional jealousy but insists he was justified in light of her infidelity. He is charming, charismatic, intuitive, but remorseful? No. An artist, a sculptor, he moulds people as creatively and deliberately as he does putty. Observing Stella's marital boredom, sensing her crazed infatuation, he plays up to it. She sees Edgar as ennobled, passing over his dreadful crime which was driven by a passion that she believes is admirable. Driven by longing and a need to punish the boredom of marriage, she later tells Peter Cleave (p. 104) that:

> she deliberately absorbed his tastes, his ideas, his feelings. His indifference to domestic comforts made her feel ashamed of all the years when the provision of domestic comfort for her husband and son had been her sole occupation.

She would later reveal to Cleave the exhilaration of the bohemian lifestyle, being a fugitive from convention, the fear of recognition, the liberation of squalor, artist and muse soaring above the drudge of housewifely routine and sexual boredom. When Cleave says she couldn't have chosen a worse character to fall for, she replies that she didn't choose, that in matters of the heart you *don't* choose.

Edgar is, in part, a myth, the 'mad artist' that works its way through literature's corridors. It's in Shakespeare as in 'the gothic', gratifying those who long for the iconic figure who stands apart from the mundane and predictable. As Johannes Gaertner (1970: 27) says: 'The artist is seen as living in opposition to society, as young, struggling, starving, arrogant, passionate in love, enjoying loose ways of living.' Thus the free-fall lifestyle, idyllic poverty and sexual licentiousness its modus operandi, cut adrift from the main and tinged with madness.

However, let's not be taken in too easily or quickly by romanticism. Actually, its very difficult to tell if as many electricians as artists experience madness but yet the artist in torment – Van Gogh amputating his ear – remains a powerful motif in Western cultural traditions, the dividing line between genius and madness seen as a narrow, even irreconcilable, fissure. Yet, whether through romanticism or professional aggrandisement, the wish to psychiatricise anything that moves should always be approached with caution.

Louis Wain (1860–1939) is a case in point. A painter of cats, he began anthropomorphising them (in postcards, calendars, children's books, etc.) placing them in different and often humorous 'human' situations. Diagnosed with schizophrenia, aged 57, he would spend his remaining fifteen years in institutions where his paintings underwent a remarkable metamorphosis. Whereas his cats were initially small and cuddly, they became scrawny and enraged, violently coloured and linearly abstract, the eyes protuberant and threatening. These changes were taken as evidence of progressive psychosis, reflecting Wain's decaying ability to impose perceptual conformity on his surroundings. However several contradictions emerge here. For instance, Wain's ability as a painter did not diminish following years of 'schizophrenia' as one would expect. This has led some to speculate that he had Asperger's syndrome where *visual agnosia* is sometimes a feature, the latter an ability to recognise the details of objects but an inability to re-represent them accurately. Who knows? Another possibility is that the cat abstractions were an expansion of Wain's vision. After all, he had, long before diagnosis, displayed cats in the most improbable, if not unpleasant, settings. Neither were the enraged cats his artistic end point, returning to his more banal images on remission from his 'schizophrenia period'. However, the point is that by widening one's focus of enquiry, more complex pictures emerge and Wain's story (Dale, 1968) is emblematic of this.

The significance of the 'psychotic gaze' is not lost in *Asylum* although it requires the traditional concept of the artist as mythic-hero. The details of Edgar's murder are gruesome but they symbolise the sculptor reshaping his material, kneading it to his liking and of course his wife had been his model. Edgar, as well, casts a dangerous shadow when contrasted with Max and this too makes sense of Stella's actions, the 'flawed hero', wounded, oppressed, confined by a boring middle-class medical mediocrity being generally attractive to women. Beyond a dutiful marriage lies sexual allure and the frisson of the illicit, in Edgar's case a deformity of sorts. For the frenzied and out of control, little notice is taken of other things. In *A Midsummer Night's Dream*, Theseus speaks:

> Lovers and madmen have such seething brains,
> Such shaping fantasies, that apprehend
> More than cool reason ever comprehends.
> The lunatic, the lover, and the poet,
> Are of imagination all compact:
> One sees more devils than vast hell can hold;
> That is, the madman; the lover, all as frantic.
>   (Act V, sc i)

Logic deserted, the world is perceived wildly, fantasy shaping reality into instability but, even if ultimately tragic, giddily preferable to the mundane.

The passion of Stella Raphael

'The history of romantic love in art and literature has been the history of adultery since the troubadours and the convention of courtly love for unattainable ladies', says A.S. Byatt (Byatt & Sodre, 2005: 205) and she's probably right. For some the 'best' sexuality is enjoyed against the prescriptions of its times. According to Samuel Hynes (1995: 316):

> passion is the necessary antagonist of convention, the protest of the individual against the rules. It is anarchic and destructive; it reveals the secrets of the heart which convention exists to conceal and repress, it knows no rules except its own necessity.

From the start, all is not well between Stella and her husband Max, albeit whether she would have continued with the marriage had she not met Stark is an open question. Sexually aroused by Edgar Stark, her devotion deepens with little notice of consequences – though she knows what these will be – socially, maritally, professionally and as a mother. As the novel proceeds, everyone with whom she makes contact comes unstuck. It's a tragedy whose underlying message is restrain passion, fight obsession, honour the rules, or pay a price.

Although psychiatry will attempt to account for Stella's behaviour, through the musings of Dr Cleave, the novel reveals psychiatry's inability to convey, even meagrely, the passions that wait on relationships like Stella and Edgar's. How to explain leaving one's comfortable middle-class existence, husband and child, to cohabit with a murderer of medieval persuasion? Behaviour like this pushes psychiatric knowledge into the unknowable, beyond the neat descriptions of a static medical practice whose models of madness are insufficient but which nevertheless possess considerable social legitimacy.

For instance, to (psychoanalytically) assert that it is not her son whom she watches drowning, but his father, fails to explain the longings for Edgar that have brought her to this point. She is hardly compulsive about any of this. There are no signs that she apprehends the anxiety that erupts when compulsion is consciously suppressed. Rather it is passion that drives her, not obsession, not compulsion: she *chooses*, wildly yes, but it's still a choice of sorts. We have heard her claim (p. 34) that she didn't choose, that in matters of the heart one doesn't, but in this she is disingenuous. In a way she has allowed her emotions to choose *for* her, to carry her towards Edgar (see p. 251). We are invited to see Edgar as a lunatic but for Stella he is a poet, a sculptor of human and inhuman forms and she has opted – despite the pinpricks of doubt – to become his willing servant.

James Joyce describes submission incomparably in Molly Bloom's soliloquy at the end of *Ulysses* (1969): as Molly lies on her bed masturbating, she says:

> I was a flower of the mountains yes when I put the rose in my hair like the Andalusian girls used or shall I wear a red yes and how he kissed me under the Moorish wall and I thought well as well him as another and then I asked him with my eyes to ask again yes and then he asked me would I yes to say yes my mountain flower and first I put my arms around him yes and drew him down to me so he could feel my breasts all perfume yes and his heart was going like mad and yes I said yes I will Yes.

Joyce called *yes* 'the female word [saying that it meant] acquiescence and the end of all resistance' (Budgen, 1960). But it is not futile resistance: it is, in Molly's case, a fierce assertion (of sexuality) and at a time and place that would warrant outrage and censure, not that, given its timelessness, that matters a damn either then or now.

What's the matter with Stella?

Why do we lie to ourselves? It's an interesting question that allows of no easy answer. McGrath (p. 17) takes us through Stella's resolve to call a halt to the liaison with Stark. She reflects that *of course* the whole thing is absurd, that it's one thing to harbour fantasies about a patient, quite another to pleasure him in public. So, at the beginning, determined to call a halt, she sets off to meet him, legs bare, lipstick on, light frock, hair brushed but, he fails to show. Later, the sordidness of their 'dance' faced up to, she establishes a more sensible and distant relationship in her mind, restoring her self-perceived role within the order of the hospital. It was a close thing but it's fine now, fine. But it isn't. She is, in fact, lying to herself at that level where each of us knows, ambivalently, that we will do that which we don't intend doing.

As matters transpire, her infatuation out of control, she goes mad at all points of the compass. Agree? No? Well then how does one weigh up mental illness if faced, on one hand, with someone diagnosed as schizophrenic and yet is relatively stable and calm, and someone whose passion is provoking chaos? Obviously she is behaving irrationally, the latter a hallmark of psychosis, inclination clouding her judgement. Having at first realised that the liaison with Edgar was wrong, somehow things have 'taken on a life of their own'. Having joined him, she soon leaves, fearing for her life only to stumble back like the proverbial child who wants picking up and putting down at the same time. In this, says Cleave (p. 27), Stella has eroticised the patient body, fetishised it perhaps being more apt. Edgar becomes a totem for the oppressed and sidelined, an idea that has fuelled every protest against conventional psychiatry through history, the psychotic as outsider, artist, dissident. The gaoler, her husband, is representative of all that is malevolent about mental health systems. Soon she will come to see Charlie as the flip side of Max and much as she will try not to, her child will become her husband's son in his attitudes as well as in his name.

Disassembling Stella

Cleave allows us to see his deconstruction of Stella (pp. 96–7). His capacity to talk and listen whilst similarly processing variables about her behaviour is fascinating. He is a class actor and as he brushes imaginary specks from immaculately pressed trousers, he never gives of himself in the relationship. He believes that at some stage prior to Charlie's death Stella sank into depression. Later, he reflects on how she must have been mad to stand idly by watching the child drown. How else to explain behaviours like these: daggers appearing before one's eyes (this volume, Chapter 9), the belief that one is an insect (this volume, Chapter 7), watching one's child drown, other than by recourse to a theory of madness? Either that or it's the more problematic 'evil', the committing of a wrongdoing that brings the priests scurrying across the fields.

Is out of control possible?

Socrates' infamous claim that no one can knowingly do wrong is apposite here. He argued that pure wisdom prevents one from doing wrong things, that evil stems from ignorance. If you know it's wrong, you won't do it. There is a horribleness to the possible truth of this. One thinks of a South African white supremacist who killed black workers by opening fire on them in a bus, later commenting that when he looked through the bus's window all he saw was animals. The moral issue is whether this guy, and those like him, are evil or mentally ill. To be mentally ill is to fit certain criteria for that and the South African didn't, unless you wish to include 'personality disorder'. That is, that he lacked a conscience, a capacity for guilt, for what he had done. But what need of conscience if he *believed* (allowing that he didn't hallucinate them as animals) that what he did was right? Perpetrators of genocide and ethnic cleansing rarely show remorse because, as they see it, they have done nothing wrong. Does it follow therefore that they are mentally ill?

For the early philosophers, habit and conditioning were high priorities in the development of virtue and the avoidance of wrongdoing. What chance does the Northern Ireland Protestant have of not hating Catholics if brought up to do precisely that? It seems that if we have not been reared with 'strength of character' then we lack the facility of knowing what separates wrong from right. Of course we can know that things are bad for us and still do them, drinking alcohol for example or smoking cigarettes. But that we always know what is morally wrong is another matter. Mass killers may know and fear the consequences of their actions but that's not quite the same as believing that they are wrong. Stella knows full well that she has cut her son adrift and watched him die and that this is wrong: but what if it is not wrong *enough*? Passion hasn't dampened her sexual urges nor did it prevent her from acting in ways highly inimical to her son's upbringing. She has a kind of moral incontinence, the worst of herself spilling over and poisoning what lives around her. She goes ahead anyway. Perhaps Socrates got it wrong.

Stella, ending up and the Medea complex

Watching Max's grim satisfaction as she suffers the consequences of her actions she charges (p. 146):

> You did this, this is your fault, he seemed always to be implying. Damn you, she thought, I shall endure this but I won't put up with this false calm of yours, this façade of neutrality and the poisonous moral superiority it masks.

It's an expression that surely speaks for the many who have endured the platitudes of orthodox psychiatry across the ages. For Stella, it is also a massive projection.

Having killed her son, albeit passively, she injects the guilt from this into her husband. It also summarises Stella's take on psychiatry since, in the second instance, she also spits her guilt at Cleave during one of their 'sessions'. Cleave takes no notice concentrating instead on an earlier projection: the Medea complex, a phenomenon in which loathing of the husband is projected onto the child. Yet Cleave then proceeds to tell us that it was not Max she saw drowning, that it was Edgar. She was killing the affair or, at base, destroying the intolerableness of her situation. Do you agree? Whose needs exactly are served by Charlie's death? Or, more precisely, by the various ways it is interpreted?

Cleave's voyeurism, his glee as he picks apart her defences, opening up her psyche, is plain. As one would dissect a frog, he tells her it was Edgar gasping in the water, that it was *his* death she saw, the termination of a calamitous love. She agrees: the longing for Stark, she says, died with Charlie, it's over. Although not for Cleave who hopes that a displacement of her feelings for Stark will take root in him as her only focus of support. Soon (p. 219) he begins to think of her as a trophy, of how good she will look amongst his living-room art, fine books and furniture. Jealous of his prey, he punishes a black-haired young patient whom he has observed watching Stella whilst lying to himself that it for his patient's good that he has done this.

Stella begins to recover. Life again comes into her as, to Cleave's satisfaction, she wakes screaming in the night. These screams, he insists, are the first stirrings of awakened humanity, a felt guilt. And yet he's unsure. She has agreed to marry him but why? He can't quite fathom her thinking and remains convinced that in some subtle way she is playing games with him. But he retains his self-satisfaction safe in the knowledge that deference is his by right. A year has passed and it is time again for the annual hospital ball. Cleave conceitedly watches as Stella, wearing a very fetching black dress, the very same that Edgar had pressed against at last year's ball, dances with various patients. Indeed, the dance goes with a swing, is a great success and all retire happily for the night.

Stella's suicide that night confirms that everything was for Edgar, every one of her moves designed to fool Cleave. There was no remorse, only a systematic duplicity whilst she hoarded enough drugs to do the trick. You may think that Cleave was spectacularly blind not to see the references to medication as a warning of potential danger. But he too had wandered from objectivity, or so he says, blind to everything except his custody of Stella as ultimate testament to his wisdom and moral prudence. As if: he knows exactly what he did and why and we get some inklings of this at the end. Cleave is in his castle and he has Edgar all to himself to play with and he has Stella's anguished, shrunken, head, sculpted by Edgar, locked in his drawer. There is no objectivity in such matters, though many psychiatrists insist there is.

Film

Directed by David Mackenzie, *Asylum* was released in 2005. Patrick McGrath is credited with writing the script with playwright Patrick Marber. It should not be confused with a horror movie of the same name released in 2008. The advertising slogan for *Asylum* was 'passion knows no boundaries'. The film was strongly cast with Ian McKellen as Cleave, Natasha Richardson as Stella, Hugh Bonneville as Max and the relatively unknown Marton Csokas as Edgar Stark.

The elements of implausibility in the novel are heightened by how the narrative of film works. Without the ambiguity of fiction it becomes even more difficult to see that someone like Stella Raphael really would fall for a murderer like Stark. That aside, the film's achievements are real enough. For example, whilst it is set in the 1950s you could be forgiven for mistaking it as Victorian and this reinforces the sense of what, but a short time ago, was a morally, especially sexually, staid world. Interesting, from Stella's viewpoint, that her husband dotes on all things Victorian, including their muffled, dutiful, marriages.

References

Altschul, A (1972) *Patient–Nurse Interaction*. London: Churchill Livingstone.

Bradbury, M (1975) *The History Man*. London: Secker and Warburg.

Budgen, F (1960) *James Joyce and the Making of Ulysses*. London: Indiana University Press.

Byatt, AS & Sodre, I (2005) Writing madness (a dialogue). In C Saunders & J Macnaughton (eds) *Madness and Creativity in Literature and Culture* (pp 202–21). Basingstoke: Palgrave Macmillan.

Clarke, L & Flanagan, T (2003) *Institutional Breakdown*. Salisbury: APS Publishing.

Dale, R (1968) *Louis Wain: The man who drew cats*. London: William Kimber.

Dryden, J (1812) *The Satires of Persius Flaccus*. London: Suttaby, Evans and Fox.

Gaertner, J (1970) Myth and pattern in the lives of artists. *Art Journal, 30(*1), 27–30.

Goffman, E (1968) *Asylums*. Harmondsworth: Penguin.

Hynes, S (1995) The epistemology of 'The Good Soldier'. In M Stannard (ed) *The Good Soldier* (pp. 310–17). London: WW Norton & Co.

Joyce, J (1969) *Ulysses*. Harmondsworth: Penguin Modern Classics.

Kakutani, M (1997) Sex with a psycho. Just for starters. *New York Times*, 14 February.

Laing, RD (1985) *Wisdom, Madness and Folly*. London: Macmillan.

Lowman, R (1997) Emerging from asylum: Freud, horror meet in the mind of McGrath. *Los Angelus Daily News*, 16 March.

McGrath, P (1997) *Asylum*. London: Penguin Books.

McWilliam, C (2000) A master of credible gothc. *Evening Standard*, 21 August.

Tonkin, B (2000) Crooked timbers of humanity. *The Independent*, 26 August.

CHAPTER 12

A QUESTION OF POWER

Torture. Something had gone wrong between sleeping and waking.
(Bessie Head)

Born in a South African mental hospital to a wealthy white woman and a black stable-hand, Bessie Head's prospects, from the first, and in every sense, were problematic. Given the racial configuration of her parents' marriage (apart from its illegality) her birth was seen as scandalous and best kept hidden. In her time South Africa was a country of race, less of people: racial status determined identity. Those of mixed race, like Bessie, were denoted 'coloured', in effect neither one thing nor the other. Bessie was eventually adopted by a 'coloured' family, an important point in both her personal and literary growth. Brought up to believe that she belonged to this family, the manner of being told, by an irate teacher, that she didn't and that her real mother was 'a lunatic' – and so she would grow up a lunatic too – deeply scarred her. In particular, she would struggle to forge these dimensions into something coherent and identifiable both in her mind and in her fiction.

Denied access to State libraries, she was given membership of a private library by an early (Indian) benefactor. A voracious reader, she now had access to the world's literature, including Hindu culture and religion, some of which figures in her work. In 1963, with her four-year-old son, she migrated to Botswana, remaining there for the rest of her life. She began to write novels, *A Question of Power* (1974) being her third, most autobiographical, most impressive. On the brink of success as a writer and no longer poor, she died from hepatitis, aged 49.

So what's it about?

It's the story of Elizabeth – Head's alter ego – who is forced to flee South Africa which is racist and oppressive. She arrives in Botswana only to find that she is an outcast there as well. Beset by persecutory delusions and lurid hallucinations occurring mainly during night-time visitations by Sello and Dan – who represent corrosive male dominance (and much more) – she continues her daily struggle to find solace in Motabeng, her adopted village. The book proceeds from Elizabeth's vantage point and is comprised of the nightly visits but with daytimes that are comparatively peaceful. In this way, two dimensions, the material and the spiritual, operate side by side:

there is a recognisable, social world of co-operative gardening, human interaction, everyday events in the village; there is also an inner, psychological constituted world, in which logic of the nightmare, and intuitive dream-association, predominates and free play of ideas is allowed to proceed.
(MacKenzie, 1999: 120–1)

It is the inner domain that interests us, how a schizophrenic tries to respond to societal hatred and the ridicule that assails her mental status as a person *and* as a female.

Opposites

The novel is about opposites. Sello and Dan are respectively the two halves of the book as well as its twin poles of black/white and male/female, their hallucinated existence also separating Elizabeth from the external world. Both are crazy for power and they lust after sex, their lack of civility towards others entirely self-centred and malevolent. Part real, part mystical, Sello inhabits a history of oppression in Africa. He is in fact all of Africa, having lived a thousand times, coming to Elizabeth in glowing monk's clothes, a veritable God: but he is also the Father of racism, the champion of caste systems. Dan, in turn, terrifies Elizabeth with his massive penis, a powerfully sexualised character whose orgies diminish women to biological recipients of male physicality. In other words, women have no voice, no opinions and no right of refusal. Both Sello and Dan (also weakly represented as persons in the real (daytime) world of Motabeng village) battle to control Elizabeth's mind and for a year she fights them. Their persecution varies, including threatening predictions about her future which, they chant, will remain in their control. The Sellos and Dans worm their way into Elizabeth's head in many guises: they stand for religion, sexuality, racism and oppression. Capricious and satanic, they come as men in suits and in religious garb, and they force her to look and listen as they inflict their abominations on her. Her struggle to deflect this allegorical intensity represents a spiritual scramble towards self-attainment. But to rid herself of them she must engage with and come to know them. So do two worlds come mesmerisingly close as when Elizabeth (p. 40) compares her hallucinatory oppressors with the power maniacs of the political present, whose attraction, she believes, lies in ordinary people's beliefs in mythology, their faith in the monstrous personalities they call 'the Gods' – but in a way that collectively leaves them open to oppression.

In terms of clinical psychiatry what is instructive here is how socio-political-racist assaults on identity can lead to psychosis, as well as how, via Elizabeth's psychosis, these attacks are construed as male-ordered both historically and contemporarily. The persecutory turbulence of this psychosis – its description – makes for a difficult read but is worth the effort both as a guide to what psychosis is like as well as the rediscovery of myth, history and culture in its genesis.

Even postcolonially, finding a language that satisfies one's masters is a humiliating endeavour. Better to confront them, but how? Franz Fanon (1986: 18) had said: 'Every colonized people – in other words, every people in whom an inferiority complex has been created by the death and burial of its local cultural originality – finds itself face to face with the language of the civilizing nation.' One means of escape is to go along, to cease being 'the Other', to join the masters (or become the new masters). For those who refuse this, the struggle will be hard because the oppression is multifaceted; history, colonialism, racism and womanhood intertwined is a perplexing mixture. Why be surprised when Elizabeth opts for a language of madness that at least articulates anguish and makes sense of the threat of the immaterial. All human suffering matters but that there may be little we can do about it warrants consideration too. Thus, again, the issue of outcomes comes to the fore but which, for the psychotic, can be little more than cruel delusion. Laing (1960: 39) puts it well:

Comprehension as an effort to reach and grasp him, while remaining within our own world and judging him by our own categories whereby he inevitably falls short, is not what the schizophrenic either wants or requires. We have to recognise all the time his distinctiveness, his separateness and loneliness and despair.

Elizabeth is all of this. That's from where the fight-back comes, from recognising power, the destructiveness of Sello and Dan and their deceptive progeny, the male-centred civilising values of the West, including its late nineteenth-century manifestation, psychiatry.

Writing madness

Women's madness is a recurrent theme in African writing. Or it may be that in such cases to be female and oppose a status quo that is heavily patriarchal must/ needs imply insanity. Commenting on this, Lillian Temu Osaki (2002) asks if 'the madwoman' is any less sane than the society that condemns her, before proceeding to the more difficult question, 'what is madness anyway?' Eschewing (Western) medical/psychological orthodoxy Osaki instead trusts writers to expose (their experiences of) insanity in black/female terms. In her view (2002: 2), what Head outlines (brilliantly) is an 'adaptation of delusion, dissociation, or other aberration to the creation of a unique view of society, her art and her own mind'.

This is some achievement because whilst it frames Head's creativity within an identifiable time and place, it also emphasises her psychological insights as, Laingian-like, her mind becomes a sanctuary from where – in the guise of her protagonist, Elizabeth – she writes herself out of madness and not just practically but conceptually and ethically as well.

Recall McGrath's contention (Ch. 2) that fiction – when dealing with madness – is about bringing lucidity to disturbance and fragmentation, a process strongly aided by traditional narrative forms. In Head's case, the writing leaps from a psyche that is little concerned with literary convention or the orthodoxies of style. This is very much an *African* account of schizophrenia dragged up from the vestiges of (an apartheid) past deeply antagonistic to black ideas and cultural assertion. Unsurprisingly, its expression is unmitigated dread, Elizabeth's nightmarish violations unsullied by literary subtleties. According to Lane (2006: 65): 'The ability to make sense of events in *A Question of Power* is always countered by the fact that the experiences of mental illness exceed sense, and refuse to be pinned down.' In writing this novel, Head could hardly, comfortably, parse thoughts into rationally segmented, accessible, bytes. Rejecting fiction's conventions she paints disturbing pictures from the authenticity of experience. She had no choice. Hers was a rough canvas to work on, necessarily revolting against (Western) approaches to clothing madness with rationality, professional interpretation and diagnosis.

Some critics take the view that Head deviates from good novel writing, that she exemplifies the unschooled in art, that what we are reading, at best, are preparatory notes or, at worst, the babblings of an unmedicated psychotic. It's no secret that many Western critics express amusement at how African novelists can sometimes foreswear (or add to) the norms of Western narrative, for instance the African novel is resented for its harangues, political declarations, bitter historical analysis and disturbing presentations of madness and the supernatural. What riles especially is the disinclination to over-fictionalise, to lighten reality's load by excluding the effects of Empire, namely political and cultural subjugation. Anozie (1972: 17) reiterates these criticisms better than most:

> No doubt the thrill of actualised prophecy can sometimes lead poets particularly in the young [i.e. black] countries to confuse their role with that of seers, and novelists to see themselves as teachers. Whatever the social, psychological, political and economic basis for it in present day Africa, this interchangeability of role between the creative writer and the prophet appears to be a specific phenomenon of underdevelopment and therefore, like it also, a passing phase.

In response, Chinua Achebe (1975) says that to talk of a people's 'level of development' is to assign (them) an immutable rung on evolution's ladder. Actually, I don't think Achebe gets this right; to me, Anozie's remarks point to African writing as *evolving* both thematically and stylistically and which in time will cease to be driven by a consciousness of deprivation. Naturally, Achebe insists that African fiction *doesn't* require further development, a development whose end point is the Europeanisation of fiction. African writing, he says, is what it is and that colonial critics:

sick and tired of Africa's 'pathetic obsession with racial cultural confrontation' should surprise no one [and that any] African who falls for this nonsense … in the face of continuing atrocities committed against millions of Africans in their land by racist minority regimes deserves a lot of pity.

(Achebe, 1975: 11)

Fair enough, but why do some African writers continue to engage with colonial issues when imperialist structures have (arguably) been dismantled? Because, the struggle against racism remains as a divisiveness bequeathed *by* imperialism, the imposition of a sociality of inferiority by white rule becoming, in turn, seminal to the afro-dictatorial, gendered, politics that followed independence. Why be surprised that this anger persistently engages African novelists? Or that it can indeed give rise to personal disintegration, consequent on rootlessness and imposed inadequacy, the essentials of colonialism's afterbirth. Head had for long failed to make sense of these connections and particularly when domiciled in apartheid South Africa. She would later reminisce:

Twenty-seven years of my life was lived in South Africa but I have been unable to record this experience in any direct way, as a writer. It is as though with all those divisions and signs, you end up with no people at all. The environment completely defeated me as a writer. I just want people to be people, so I had no way of welding all the people together into a cohesive whole.

(Driver, 1993: 165–6)

She thought life would be different in Botswana as her early fiction shows. But in *A Question of Power* she realises that cruelty and dispossession are unconfined by geography. In fact, the move to Botswana turned out to be another painful dislocation for Bessie, although it did push her into writing partly through felt anger but also from deep inside her developing psychosis.

Black radicalism

But cruelty is not all. As Bessie knew, what counted as madness in Western psychiatry was, at the time, subject to an emergent critique which saw it as Eurocentric and patronising. Head's novel is intrinsic to that critique, deploying, as intellectual ballast, Fanon's (1986) discourse on psychiatry's stereotyping African people as evil and mad. In Elizabeth, Head *personifies* statelessness, fractured identity, and an awareness of the role played by the dual enmities of myth and rationality. In this, Elisabeth expresses the emotionality of madness that complements Fanon's intellectual disputation. Discussing madness in 'the black,' Fanon (1986: 145) states that:

we have to fall back on the idea of *collective catharsis* [original italics]. In every society, in every collectivity, exists – must exist – a channel, an outlet through which the forces accumulated in the form of aggression can be released.

The problem is that colonial literature denoted 'the black' as primitive, uncultured, with the white missionary a bringer of reason but more so, a saviour of the heathen soul. Homi Bhabha, in his introduction, 'Remembering Fanon' (Fanon, 1986), said that colonialism deeply disturbs 'the social and psychic representation of the human subject', that 'humanity becomes estranged within the colonial condition' collapsing in on itself in bits and pieces. In the following extract from Fanon – which Bhabba calls 'an agonising performance of self-images' – and which bristles inside Head's prose – we read (1986: xii):

> I had to meet the white man's eyes. An unfamiliar weight burdened me. In the white world the man of colour encounters difficulties in the development of his bodily schema ... I was battered down by tom toms, cannibalism, intellectual deficiency, fetishism, racial defects ... I took myself far off from my own presence. What else could it be for me but an amputation, an excision, a haemorrhage that spattered my whole body with black blood.

These words are from a psychiatrist, not a psychotic, yet they bestow dignity, as well as accuracy, on the process of 'taking one's self off from a presence' constituted (by others) in derogatory and oppressive terms. Fanon's protest however stems from a revolutionary dissention from a racially elitist medical system. Head had learned from this insofar as she absorbed Fanon's points of reference, his articulation of dissent from a medical framework which subsumes and sorts distress into illnesses. This, in effect, remains the role that orthodox psychiatry plays in our lives now, arbitrating between the outside and the internal worlds of people in diagnostic terms.

Radical psychiatry

A fault line of radical psychiatry was that it romanticised schizophrenia as a means of insight into human nature generally or as something which provoked creativity, or both. R.D. Laing had likened schizophrenia to a heroic voyage and although we reject this now, the contemporary assertion that hearing voices can be beneficial (to patients) also idealises psychotic experience. We've witnessed how Head's novel drew from radical psychiatry so it hardly surprises that she too is blamed for trumpeting insanity's would-be 'healing function'. Says Joanne Chase (1982: 74):

> Bessie Head does not skimp on the ugliness of insanity, but yet it seems a misrepresentation of the ordeal of the mentally ill to claim that it is creative

and productive rather than simply a sickness like any other. The book enters the realm of fantasy and romance in its implication that only an irrational, visionary experience can lead to insight, rather than the hard spade work of the intellect.

In particular, the switch into regeneration, at the novel's end, is too quick, too easy and takes place with too little warning. And yet why be sceptical about this? Well, because orthodox psychiatry denotes illness in ABC terms, with recovery nine-tenths an outcome of 'interventions', patients as passive recipients of drugs and psychotherapies. Head counters this, showing that any recovery that excludes catharsis, that is expressed as *outcomes,* is inadequate. The fact is, most professional accounts of psychiatric distress are formulaic, tending to present patients:

> in terms of their diagnoses, with everything else in their lives reduced to evidence in support of that claim. The patient's arrival at the hospital is the climactic moment in many physician's accounts, with the progress of the treatment the central plot.
> (Hornstein, 2002: 8)

And the problem with this is that it sits uneasily with distress that comes from existential angst where 'expectations of outcome' only add to the problem. Combine this with the psychological anguish associated with economic depression and matters dramatically alter in terms of what can be achievable as 'results'. To oppose mainstream psychiatry, however, is to risk accusations of romanticism, of denying 'evidence-based' practice, of challenging the idea of mental illness as biologically based or as an error of learning. This is unfair insofar as radical psychiatry never did this: what it did do was censure the institutionalising of behaviour and practice that inevitably accompanies such thinking. It damned an approach to mental distress whose premise was that people possess inherent flaws (or learn them) and that when 'those flawed' are corralled this promotes pessimism and an ambiance of inactivity.

Critiquing the supposed idealism in *A Question of Power*, Driver (1993: 168) says:

> The text's affirmative ending – which reads more like an act of will than an organically conceived resolution – is again constructed around the sense of community, which (appropriately to Head's general project) is emphatically placed as vision rather than reality: [falling asleep, Margaret] placed one soft hand over her hand. It was a gesture of belonging.

But Head's novel is about how communities cohere around mythical/ transcendental icons, her culture's endemic means of coping (and surviving) its residual and ongoing problems. Less interested in medicine's claims about what ails Elizabeth, Head seeks an explanation of how social/gendered/spiritual factors, now and in history, translate into helping people work through their distress. Ultimately a quantum of solace comes from tilling the land. This is a powerful motif in any agrarian community, land as maternal, the provider of sustenance and regeneration. We in the West have perhaps mislaid Fanon's contention that 'the social' is a plethora of unresolved power plays existing alongside individual suppressions of desire and need. We blandly watch clinical psychiatry as it homogenises different groups, some of them culturally oppressed, into the belief that words such as delusion and 'acting out' actually possess meaning to them, when actually they are merely a method of defining insanity in the most trivial of ways.

To an extent, the representation of 'Sixties Radical Psychiatry' has been a lie. Entirely misogynist and unable/unwilling to shift the diagnostic framework entirely it quickly retreated into protestations by individuals – R.D. Laing, David Cooper – unable to form a coherent response to orthodoxy. In fairness, it hardly falls to radicalism to do that but, as Laing acknowledged, he lacked the talent to formulate a therapeutic strategy that gathered in the social and political as well as the existentialist. Of course *radicalism* had some positive effects albeit intellectual iconoclasm beached it from the everyday needs and requirements of most mentally distressed people. Like psychoanalysis, it would eventually make its presence felt more productively in literature and the arts generally.

The details of oppression

A crux of the novel is the Principal of Elizabeth's Mission School telling her to:

> be very careful. Your mother was insane. If you're not careful you'll get insane just like your mother. You're mother was a white woman. They had to lock her up, as she was having a child by a stable boy, who was a native.
> (p. 16)

Elizabeth concludes that the Principal must be: 'the last, possibly, of the kind who had heard "the call" from Jesus and come out to save the heathen' (p. 16) but she knows that 'the call' rarely stirs 'the kind' to protect those for whom they profess to care. Initially, the Principal's hypocrisy elicits only hate, but then Elizabeth begins to: 'wonder if the persecution had been so much the outcome of the Principal's twisted version of life as the silent appeal to her dead mother' (p. 17) who calls to her from beyond the grave: 'Now you know. Do you think I can bear the stigma of insanity alone? Share it with me' (p. 17). This is madness pulled from memory, the ancients revisiting the present, making bridges between human distress and its origins. Children, confronted with expressions of parental distress, not infrequently introject this guiltily. It's as if they seek a share in the distress, or experience responsibility for it. These are the psychological explanations mental health professionals favour. However, African ancestry invokes transcendence as more than mere explanation, it intuits causative influences upon the warp and weft of a person's madness. At this point a paradox shows itself in Head's insistence that hers was a literature of universal significance. It was not an African, feminist or any other type of book. As she put it: 'It's not so much a question of being black as of having got control of life's learning' (in Driver, 1993: 176).

We discover (Head 1974: 132–7) that Elizabeth rejects the tenets of 'black power' with its images of raised black-gloved fists: 'it seems an indignity to me' she says, 'I couldn't do it, I'd feel ashamed' and when asked why, she responds: 'because of what I see inside, because of what I'm learning internally'. This is a transformative novel, not in the way of superficial slogans or protestations but through inculcating spirituality and traditions that stem from a consciousness of communal tradition. Through a narrative of extreme intensity, turning within and without itself with serpentine ease, madness is now representative of history and the regenerative powers of people working the land together. In this, Head plays her trump card, the psychotic imagination resisting its shadowy negative, talking back to a millennia of victimisation.

A note about the biological

Lane (2006: 69) draws on Maithufi (1997) to insinuate that Head, like Fanon, confuses a biology of race with ideology, that they position blackness as a configuration of identity, ignoring how concepts of 'self' entail a psychology that is individual and social. In effect, emphasising race confirms white imperialist designations of 'the Black' or 'Asian' or 'Irish' as 'Other'. The fact is, superiority and inferiority are products of ideological *intention*, political constructs designed to attach negative qualities to different groups on grounds that are always iniquitous. Crossed wires are possible here inasmuch as Bessie's novel deconstructs gender and race against conflicting theories of madness. Her view is not that blackness is a causative factor but how colonised groups view themselves from an externally *imposed* inferiority. Head's opposition to this is to posit mental illness as a pivot upon which to draw upon a black mythology. No longer a passive receptacle for Sello's historical pageants or Dan's pornography, Elizabeth calls on themes of gentility and faith in people all told. We smell her sweat as she grasps at the straws of sanity, witness the eerie remembrances that ignite her night-time reveries. Like all nightmares they're beyond rationalisation yet weirdly recognisable.

Myth and sex

Initially, Elizabeth invests Sello and Dan with immense power. Their night-time visitations are rivetingly described in the Dan section of the book (pp. 103–5). In particular, the phantasmagorical changing of matter to non-matter, unremitting transmogrifications of air, wind and fire into humanoid forms, are sinisterly frightening. She recalls (p. 107) a headless woman, a gruesome figure in a long black dress who:

> had slowly walked into [her]. She underwent a transformation during the night, and at dawn she emerged from Elizabeth's chest area, in a burst of golden yellow light. She had found her head again and was dressed in soft, sun-yellow dress.

What's remarkable is that although caught up in this medieval horror she remains lucid, capable of real-world relationships. There is a message here. No one is ever fully mad, no one is ever beyond the pale of communication (however odd they sound), nobody ceases to love or need respect. *A Question of Power* comes from a psychosis lashed with hallucination and dread but somehow fulfilling a promise of hope and engagement.

Few can doubt that Elizabeth – and Bessie Head too – experienced what is commonly called paranoid schizophrenia. But in both cases it's a psychosis steeped in histories and cultures and now stained with the terror of totalitarianism. For Elizabeth, to be 'coloured' was to be ill, forced to live with a nervous tension, because you: 'did not know why white people had to go out of their way to hate you … they were just born that way, hating people, and a black man or woman was just born to be hated'. The novel's tension stems from delusions which are formed from the fractured societies in which Elizabeth must live. Hers is the struggle of black Africa in which her individuality, quashed by racism and dictatorship, gains release through fiction that opposes what has and is being done to her. Of course we can't know if the story's hallucinatory segments come from Head's psychosis but we may suppose so. Certainly the night-time segments stem from madness, the daytime 'realities' forming an opposing tension intended to inform readers but, as well, to intensify the horrors of the dark. Few people prefer dark to light. Jung (1938) teaches that the dark comprises the shadows of the unconscious and we generally fear this in a paradoxical way that includes being freed from it. Head places psychosis at its most vulnerable during the night, possibly because 'blackness' generally she equates with oppression. One thinks of someone: 'cast into darkness' the genesis of the outcaste being a fall from grace, a falling away from the light. She however sees this 'soul darkness' as transitory and redemptive because it is not inherent but imposed. As such, you have to fight to recover, regenerate every fibre in your being as the means to a better end.

Recovery and the garden

Many of you may be too young to remember that the old hospitals/asylums had farms and gardens providing opportunities for patients to till the soil, to make things grow, to reconnect with practical demands and realities. Of course we needed to close these institutions but how noticeable that even the desultory attempts to retain 'the garden' in community-based settings has become defunct. We seem to have reinvented a psychiatry composed of pharmacology and psychological techniques, a martinet profession bereft of much social, cultural or ethnic process. And yet there is good evidence that people benefit from physical exercise and 'the outdoors' in terms of mental well-being.

In 2005, BBC News reported that Dundee University had conducted a three-year review of gardening projects, finding them beneficial to people's mental health both personally and, as well, in terms of integrating people into the wider community. Health Minster Edwina Hart (Brindley, 2008) said about a similar project in Wales: 'patients and staff have gained enormously from the development' and not just in terms of growing food but by using the spaces the gardens provide, as well as the reciprocity that such undertakings demand particularly if linked to economic gain. For Elizabeth and the people of Motabeng, working the garden and ensuring its productivity becomes a healing factor because their co-operative, and others, epitomises their nation. To get to this communal position Elizabeth has endured a purgatory on earth, lacerated by monstrous patriarchies that have nearly destroyed her. Her scream (p. 14) that to cohabitate with men is like: 'a clear sensation of living life inside a stinking toilet' is the opposite of the good earth, signifying what is putrid, dead, bunged up: 'How had she fallen so low? It was a state below animal, below living and so dark and forlorn no loneliness and misery could be its equivalent' (p. 14).

Green is an overused word these days but its credentials remain strong, its potential as a catalyst for human development significant. Although lulled into a therapeutic hibernation it seems now, given the rise of what is (eclectically) called 'care farming', that the uses of gardening and farm work can be reaffirmed. Of course we need to avoid the faux romanticism of returning to 'the good life', of recreation for its own sake. Therapies based on a green environment must be thought through and organised to some purpose. Discussing the pros and cons of ecotherapy Burls (2008: 234) says that it:

> provides concrete examples of the consequences associated with individual and group action. Giving insights into any change which may occur in the natural environment and providing the relevant guide for metaphors. Aiding experiential, narrative and curative learning, providing the backdrop and time for individual reflection, modelling, self disclosure, and metaphoric processing.

To which one can add the wider consciousness of community, belonging and ownership. There have to be many people for whom 'the land', the notion of growth and nurturance, is fundamental and I believe that ecotherapy groups ignited by the potential benefits of mutual work will spread and acquire respect. In the light of competing therapies this will need to be researched albeit, given its nature, without recourse to the so-called 'gold standard' of the randomised controlled trial (RCT). Perhaps we need to substitute 'green standard' as a more appropriate way forward. Of course it will take a lot to shift the social standing of RCTs since we seem to have disposed of human testimony as a defensible measure of outcomes. This poses a dilemma for researchers, to forgo the RCT risks the prospect of client's narratives being derided as anecdotal. This is why Bessie Head's novel is such an impressive contribution, the proof is in the reading of it and hundreds of thousands have, although sadly not from within the 'helping professions'.

In combating Sello she was up against the histories of Africa and the wisdom of the ages. In addition, Dan has bludgeoned her with his conglomerates of sex, race, religion and political dogma. The subjugators of females, Sello and Dan are mad destroyers complementing one another as they slurp up one inflicted degradation after another. That Sello and Dan might uncover the links between madness and power, 'whether in her dubious sanity or in the strangeness of the men themselves' (p. 19) there is no doubting their hatred of Elizabeth. Ultimately their antics lead to her salvation because in refusing to fight them *with violence* she avoids becoming like them. This is because, finally, she sees them for what they are and in opting for charity she *chooses* not to remain insane. But in this we are asked, possibly naïvely, to believe that a love (of mankind) is a sufficient weapon against madness. 'I could not grasp the darkness because at the same time I saw the light' (p. 190) is what made her 'live with' Sello and Dan for so long. Release comes suddenly when Tom (p. 188) laughingly tells her that love is for both people and vegetables:

> Her soul death was really over in that instant, though she did not realise it. He seemed to have, in an intangible way seen her sitting inside that coffin, reached down and pulled her out. The rest she did herself. She was poised from that moment to make the great leap out of hell.

At every level, how to cope with male violence is pertinent: does one ape traditional, male-oriented, styles of action or try to find alternatives. In 'They've found *another* way to hurt us' (Clarke, 1988), a woman inmate in a forensic unit describes how 'control and restraint' – by whatever euphemism this is now known – becomes an exercise in physical disablement, often painfully inflicted on young females deemed: 'borderline personality disorder'. The latter too euphemises perceived badness in women and whose persistent objections and resistance are responded to with autocracy and physical/mental immobilisation. The problems of psychiatry and gender remain, as much an outcome of their being ignored and under-discussed as anything else.

Not that Head (p. 70) provides easy answers either. 'What is Love?', she asks, 'Who is God? If I cry, who will have compassion on me as my suffering is the suffering of others? This is the nature of evil. This is the nature of goodness.' Perhaps being unable to separate one's self from others is why the novel's two worlds are at odds, but more so is it the schizoid inability to choose between the internal and external. As Laing (1960: 94) observed – in a commentary with surprising behaviourist overtones:

> the tendency of the individual to place itself beyond the threat of reality only serves to perpetuate the superiority of that reality against a weaker self: to participate in life is only possible therefore through anxiety and existential dread and the tolerance thereof. Franz Kafka knew this very well, when he said that it was only through his anxiety that he could participate in life, and, for this reason, he would not be without it.

A note on colonial psychiatry

Over fifty years ago 'the African' (Carothers, 1951: 14) was described in a *Journal of Mental Science* article as someone who failed: 'to recognise the intrinsic nature of cause and effect. He possesses a certain amount of knowledge of nature but for the greater part it is pseudo-science, knowledge mixed with a child-like play of the imagination.' It was this same article – fully 'substantiated' by leading psychiatric figures at the time – that excused 'the African' from psychiatric diagnosis on grounds that he/she was too simple of mind, his/her culture too primitive and childlike to succumb to such morbid states. Except in one instance, which Carothers (1951: 21) took pains to note:

> Largely determined by his passing emotions, he does lack foresight, perseverance and sustained determination, he does evince a keen intuitive empathy and a corresponding disregard for truth, his unreliability and irresponsibility are notorious from a European standpoint, his ability to learn from experience and adapt to reality is very variable, and his lack of judgement and faulty synthesis [are] apparent.

So he lacks the complexity necessary for psychosis but which is not required for psychopathy. In other words, potentially he's dangerous.

Later reports (Orley & Wing, 1979) would contradict Carothers' general findings, reporting instead indices of female depression at least as high, if not higher, than some British samples. Interestingly, Brown and Harris's (1978) seminal *Social Origins of Depression* had contemporarily highlighted the role of social factors in the evolution of depression in British women. Orley and

Wing (1979), however, played this down in their Ugandan studies, denying: 'a linear relationship between severity of depression and the number and severity of adverse experiences'. Even in this reasonably careful study, the limited emphasis on the effects of hostile environments was sustained as were various inferences of the researchers, the chief investigator, for instance, being white.

Although much has changed since, it is worth noting how orthodox psychiatry, whilst reacting moderately to radical psychiatry's critique – there were some positive reviews of Laing's work in mainstream journals – when this critique turned its gaze on the negative outcomes of psychiatry in non-European countries it was generally ignored. One thinks again of Fanon's (1986) *Black Skin, White Masks* which remained all but unnoticed for years and continues to be derided by some.

Universality

My third novel, *A Question of Power*, had such an intensely personal and private dialogue that I can hardly place it in the context of the more social and outward looking work I had done. It was a private philosophical journey to the sources of evil.
(Head, 1990: 69)

However the personal *is* the universal insofar as, in this story, socio-political degradations become an obvious backcloth to Elizabeth's struggles. The fact is, allegorical novels purvey political ends and *A Question of Power* is no exception given that its big issue, as its title tells us, is power, power that obstructs the human spirit in its desire to unite people in caring and ethically good ways. Movements such as therapeutic communities and service user groups smack of this, of people finding solace and truth with one another's shared experiences. Sadly, much of mental health stands colonised by therapists and their endless mantra of 'the evidence base'. I would like to propose that *A Question of Power* be incorporated into the family of evidences: its anxio-mythic account of mental suffering and recovery a needed lesson for us all.

References

Achebe, C (1975) *Morning Yet on Creation Day*. London: Heinemann.

Anozie, S (1972) *Christopher Okigbo*. London: Evans Brothers.

BBC News (2005) Garden theory over mental health. 30 May. Online: Available; *http://news.bbc.co.uk/1/hi/scotland/4587625.stm*

Brindley, M (2008) Garden for mental health patients at St Tydfil's Hospital. November 14. Online: Online: Available; *http://www.walesonline.co.uk/news/cardiff-news/2008/11/14/garden-for-mental-health*

Brown, GW & Harris, T (1978) *Social Origins of Depression*. London: Tavistock.

Burls, AP (2008) Seeking nature: A contemporary therapeutic environment. *Therapeutic Communities, 29* (3), 228–44.

Carothers, JC (1951) Frontal lobe function and the African. *Journal of Mental Science, 97*, 12–48.

Chase, J (1982) Bessie Head's 'A Question of Power': Romance or rhetoric? *ACLALS Bulletin, 72*, 74–5.

Clarke, L (1988) They've found *another* way to hurt us. *Changes, 6 (2)*, 54–6.

Driver, D (1993) Reconstructing the past, shaping the future: Bessie Head and the question of feminism in a new South Africa. In G Wisker (ed), *Black Women's Writing* (pp 160–87). Basingstoke: Macmillan.

Fanon, F (1986) *Black Skin, White Masks*. New York: Grove Press.

Head, B (1974) *A Question of Power*. London: Heinemann.

Head, B (1990) *A Woman Alone: Autobiographical writings*. Portsmouth, NH: Heinemann.

Hornstein, GA (2002) Narratives of madness, as told from within. *The Chronicle Review*, 25 January issue, 7–10.

Jung, CG (1938) *Psychology and Religion*. New Haven, CT: Yale University Press.

Lane, RJ (2006) *The Postcolonial Novel*. Cambridge: Polity Press.

Laing, RD (1960) *The Divided Self*. London: Tavistock.

MacKenzie, C (1999) *Bessie Head*. New York: Twayne Publishers.

Maithufi, S (1997) Fanon's African ontology, postcolonial-ideological stage and the liberation of Africa. APA Newsletter. Available online at: www.apaonline.org/publications/newsletters/v97n1_Black_05.aspx

Orley, J & Wing, JK (1979) Psychiatric disorders in two African Villages. *Archives of General Psychiatry, 36*, 513–20.

Osaki, LT (2002) Madness in black women's writing. *The Ahfad Journal, 19* (1), 4–20.

CHAPTER 13

THE GOOD SOLDIER

The lamps are going out all over Europe; we shall not see them lit again in our lifetime.
(Viscount Edward Grey)

The author of *The Good Soldier*, Ford Madox Ford (1915/1995), believed that novels should be realist, that it was important to attribute motives and beliefs to characters so as to underpin their actions and movements, the very elements that make for 'a good read'. What matters in fiction, said Ford, is the extent to which characters account their position in historical terms and developmentally. But note, as well, that his characters are not just strongly written, but written as types, for example as Catholic or Protestant. Witness John Dowell's take (pp. 46–7) on English Catholics as a people grounded in 'strong cold conscience' with the Continental (and Irish) variety 'a dirty, jovial and unscrupulous crew'. As we shall see, there are reasons for these sweeping inferences.

However, as *The Good Soldier* proceeds, generalisations, even characterisation itself, begins to lose its persuasion and in the case of Dowell, the narrator, one realises that all is not what it seems. Levenson (2004: 106–7), for instance, notes how Dowell:

> begins with the presuppositions typical of much Victorian characterisation: the individual conditioned by circumstance, composed of intelligible motives, susceptible to moral analysis, the justified self. Then ... he moves to a conception of character beyond the reach of social explanation.

Such as into instinct for instance, or passion or unpredictability, themes of human primitiveness that evade conventional storytelling. Just as musical sound can be warped in pursuance of emotional effect, so does Ford twist traditional narrative such that it becomes unstable, improbable, and untrustworthy. What transpires is a mosaic of traits, dimensions, expressions to which *we* impose meanings so as to make sense of it all. As such, if you're looking for a 'good read', *The Good Soldier* is no easy romp. Ford, for instance, doesn't let Dowell in on the full story: he is allowed to tell the story, but without complete knowledge of it at any given time. Generally, with novels, one relies on the narrator to reveal all, almost as though he is the writer's agent. Not in this case where Dowell not only sees what's around him dimly, slowly, but also with assumptions that people are inherently good, socially obligated and trustworthy, a comfort zone brought about through blind faith in humanity. But behind the faces of 'the good people' lurks that which is undesirable: infidelity, betrayal, passion, suicide, madness and the impoverishment of a class whose grand houses are mere Disneyland, appearance without depth.

Eventually, Dowell will venture behind the façade of social fraternity and show us the underbelly of the novel's characters. Via an ambitious use of 'the unreliable narrator' he will laboriously excavate the motives that underlie behaviour and it is this which makes *The Good Soldier* a masterwork of human psychology. Eschewing a traditional (but false) linear unscrambling of 'events', it researches the unconscious of its characters. In this, it is not just a tale of four people going about their business, but a rendition of the intrapersonal psychology of two couples caught within a matrix of diminishing awareness and a vanishing way of life.

So what is it about?

Well it seems straightforward, at first. In 1904 two couples, the Dowells (John and Florence), Americans, and the Ashburnhams (Edward and Leonora), English, meet whilst 'taking the waters' at Nauheim, a health spa in Germany. They go there each year because both Florence Dowell and Edward Ashburnham have heart conditions *or so it appears*. Edward, by the way, is 'the good soldier', named as such by Dowell, our unreliable narrator. Wealthy, from an old Philadelphian family, Dowell has a well-intentioned faith in the world as it presents itself, as well as a Shakespearean commitment to social order. To the point of absurdity, he cannot pierce the surface of persons: unable to see people 'warts and all' he invests them with prodigious trust and propriety. Never was the Kantian dictum: 'we see things not as they are but as we are' more apposite. However, in Dowell's case there is the added complicatedness of his psychological blandness. As Smiley (2006: 8) puts it: 'The narration has the sense of being an unravelling of what has happened via the interpretation of someone who would in fact rather not have known.'

And yet, says Meixner (1962: 320):

> Ford has created one of the most remarkable, one of the most subtle characterisations ... almost completely from within he has caught and rendered the sensibility of a severely neurotic personality. He is a man who, incapable of acting, is almost entirely feeling, a creature of pure pathos.

And so not the best person to render a complex story even-handedly. Narration, if to be accessible, needs a storyteller who can at least enlighten us via the straightforwardness of events as perceived by him. Who needs the murky distillations of neurotic, divided, men or women when living can be rendered more comfortably, more simplistically. Not Ford Madox Ford who considered the straightforward a derogation of truth, his narration seeking to show people in duplicitous and unpredictable guises.

We have already seen how, at the time, [*The Good Soldier* was first published in 1915] artists were increasingly preoccupied with double lives. Irish novelist Colm Tóibin identifies the motivation for dualism as the thrill of secrecy but whose other side is the desire to be found out. Whether as the (usually evil) alter ego of an upright man or as a revelation from the repressed shadow of an unconscious it works itself around the undergrowth of coordinated civility. From first meeting, the couples become friends with Dowell affirming Edward's moral worth, a noble character in whom one could place an infinite trust. But behind Dowell's back, and for twelve years, Edward has been sleeping with his wife: it seems he is not so trustworthy after all! Nor is this his first extramarital assignation, he has betrayed Leonora before. Thus is adulterous marriage centrifugal in unravelling the narrative's secrets to its participants and to us. But that comes later. To begin with, we have a couple of couples living the high life in Europe, taking the medicinal waters, visiting the cultural hot spots whilst being waited on 'hand and foot'. Theirs is, self-consciously, a superior way of life, witness the aforementioned exclusion of continentals, Catholics, and Irish as social pariahs. This was indeed, at the time, the 'charmed life' of people from 'above stairs' and which would vanish with the coming of the Great War (1914–18) that prompted Edward Grey's observation that the lights of Europe were going out forever. We shall follow this story to its end. For the moment, Edward is having sex with Florence. Edward's wife knows this, Dowell doesn't. Further, Dowell has never had sex with Florence, whose 'heart condition' forbids it. Not that Edward and Leonora are up front either: outwardly civil, they have not spoken in private for thirteen years.

What kind of novel?

It's pretty unique in terms of narration. 'Ford [had] remarked that the novel had always gone "straight forward" in its apprehension of character; whereas in real life you never go straight forward, but obliquely, or round about' (Trotter, 2001: 211). When W.C. Fields remarked of Mae West that she 'came at him in sections' he wasn't referring to just her curves. In other words, we discover who people are in fits and starts, haphazardly, by chance. The man you thought highly dependable turns out to be risky with others' money; a stickler for the social proprieties carries a criminal past or lives a disreputable present. To get a handle on people means working around their idiosyncrasies and contradictions and with a keen ear for what may initially seem inconsequential but which turns out not to be. Kingsley Amis (1992: 99) recalls a reunion that laid bare some disappointing truths:

It was more dismal to realise that I had not looked at any of them closely enough before, had seen only superficial differences where there were real substantial ones, had missed the fact that Signalman X and Driver Y were amiable bores while Corporal Hazel was lively, amusing, to be listened to. And, oh God, we do that all the time, go through life not properly noticing people or valuing them as they deserve. Not even those we love? A large scotch please.

Amis's summation is a tad depressive and possibly self-serving. That is, he seems to say why try too hard, when you can always agonise over it later. *The Good Soldier* however holds out some confidence in our capacity to apprehend the past's meanings in terms of the present.

> Ford emphasises how states of affairs are given to us with an inherent incompleteness that we strive to complete. Similarly, by scattering the elements of Dowell's history across the course of his narrative, Ford calls attention to how understanding depends on consistency building.
> (Armstrong, 1987: 206)

And not just Dowell but we too as we try to make sense of things. Ford was one of the first novelists to experiment with time, more or less pioneering the use of flashback and forward, even leaving spaces along the way for readers to conjecture events this way and that. It's fascinating because it does mirror how we gauge people and events across time. Ford invites us to impose coherence on fleeting events and the multiple impressions that attend them. The point is not that the narrative is disjointed as much as that we are made party to how it is made sense of and why this matters *in* the novel. This is an unstable world, indeterminism leading to indecision, deception. In its opening pages, both couples are so in tune that Dowell likens them to an exquisitely danced minuet. However, within six or so pages he retrospectively tells (p. 12) us that:

> It wasn't a minuet that we stepped; it was a prison – a prison full of screaming hysterics … and yet, I swear … it was true. It was true sunshine; the true music; the true splash of the fountains from the mouth of stone dolphins. For, if for me we were four people with the same tastes, with the same desires, acting – or no not acting – sitting here and there unanimously, isn't that the truth? If for nine years I have possessed a goodly apple that is rotten at the core and discover its rottenness only in nine years and six months less four days, isn't it true to say that for nine years I possessed a goodly apple?

Thus the challenge is to understand what *underlies* appearance. Neither Florence, Edward nor Leonora are what they seem. No one is. Marriage particularly takes a hammering. Stripped of love, loyalty and fidelity, it retains mainly a potential to control. For example, infidelity provides Edward with the comforts that stem from the controlling influence of Leonora. And when Dowell affects shock on discovering marital disloyalty it is not the sexual elements that disturb as much as the belief (p. 15) that:

> If everything is so nebulous about a matter so elementary as the morals of sex, what is there to guide us in the more subtle morality of all other personal contacts, associations, and activities? Or are we meant to act on impulse alone? It is all darkness.

From this comes the tendency to create order, to categorise people and ideas, rearguard actions of control and safety. So, for Dowell, are there Catholics of this type and that, as well as normal and abnormal, passion and restraint. For years, Dowell has seen the world a certain way, his way. That the social order is mere chimera and not the 'reality' he believes it to be passes him by. A servant to his wife, he can't for the life of him work out how she slept with Edward Ashburton (p. 12).

> I don't believe that for one minute she was out of my sight, except when she was safely tucked up in bed and I downstairs, talking to some good fellow or other in some lounge or smoking room.

But even 'the smoking room' befuddles him. Gentlemen with urbane and civilised faces telling smutty jokes, England's finest who would defend, in other circles, womanly virtue to the death, women of his class that is, of similar birthright. But not Edward Ashburnam. Dowell reminisces how such a man was loathe to indulge in lascivious talk, a man of noble caste given to doing good by the poor: 'exactly the sort of chap you could trust your wife with. And I trusted mine and it was madness' (p. 14). But what of Dowell himself? Examining his conscience, he finds it clean. Never having as much as *inclined* towards impropriety, he remains confident in the spotlessness of his thoughts, his chastity. What does this make him? Some kind of secular saint I suppose, provided of course *you believe him.*

Reality's bites

The Good Soldier questions the dependability of perception and reality formation from the first with Dowell confusedly disclaiming (p. 15):

> I don't know how best to put this down – whether it would be right to try and tell the story from the beginning, as if it were a story; or whether to tell it from this distance of time, as it reached me from the lips of Leonora.

Talk about Chinese whispers. Forsooth, the novel's opening line: 'This is the saddest story I have ever heard', pronounces the story *already told*. That is, it's in the telling that its characters come alive, including for he who tells it but who has already heard it from someone else. This is making life up in the living of it and largely by imposing categories of etiquette that reflect a need to maintain order.

The point about categories is supported from psychosociological research. Harold Garfinkel (1967) demonstrated how people 'author', 'document', or 'authenticate' their lives when encountering others. Like Goffman (1990) Garfinkel doesn't presuppose an ordered world: social order is fictitious, chaotic, and the job of persons, consciously or otherwise, is to construct realities from it, to scrutinise, assimilate and reassemble events that make autobiographical sense. Garfinkel suggests that we do this irrespective of the veracity of what is observed.

To assess this he constructed a test whereby university students presented emotional problems to a psychotherapist pre-programmed to respond 'yes' or 'no' [in the sense of 'yes' indicating a positive and 'no' a negative response in general terms]. In addition, the 'yes' or 'no' option is chosen not by evaluating the student's issues but according to random number. That is, the student relates a problem, a random number is flashed to a therapist who provides, in general terms, a positive or negative response. Garfinkel's findings were that whatever the response, students strove to make sense of it, even when the information given was contradictory. When, for instance, a student repeated a question or added a supernumerary they stood a statistically equal chance of receiving a different answer. So if the question: 'you think I should leave my girlfriend?' initially elicited a 'no' and where the follow-up: 'You *really* think I should leave her?' obtained a 'yes', this didn't prevent a student rationalising what was being said.

Context is important here: the psychotherapeutic encounter exerts disproportionate power on those who seek its wisdom and whilst not clinically ill, these students were psychologically vulnerable. Vulnerability *invites* the comfort (even of strangers), disposing itself towards solutions however unlikely they be. True, Garfinkel's results may simply reflect a mannered version of 'clutching at straws' for people either uncomfortable with life or whose needs are difficult to articulate.

This is the case with John Dowell whose assumptions are fatally undermined and whose role is to interpret and communicate how and why this has happened. But having premised a moral order on solidity and endurance, he slowly recognises that he, and his kind, *don't* comprise an external (elevated) orderliness, that values and beliefs are contingent on drive, deceit and lust. So a world comes apart but without precluding its starting up again, albeit differently, and it is this that the novel explores. But how? For a start, Dowell occupies centre stage and it becomes difficult not to accept his version of events. To all intents and purposes he is 'Garfinkel's psychotherapist' and by means of his testimony we, 'his students', impose order on or make sense of things. Unlike Garfinkel's experiment, though, Dowell (ultimately) reveals himself as a charlatan whose descriptions are misleading, the story having run rings around its characters, us, and time. 'Time waits for no man', says the proverb: onwards we go, grappling with the 'slings and arrows of outrageous fortune', often with no time to look back whether in anger or in certainty. Nevertheless, Dowell's flitting backwards and forwards, although disruptive, lets us see events from multiple, illuminative, points. The indeterminedness and narrative uncertainty are also minimised by psychological mechanisms – Heider's (1958) Attribution Theory for example – that also filters ambiguity as part of the construction of precepts and events.

Beyond psychology

However, though psychology informs us, my concern is to show how literature, in this instance *The Good Soldier*, builds upon its ideas. For instance, the novel's repressive elements insinuate the potential of an eventful future, progression and regression constantly hitting off one another. Hynes (1995) says that in story-type novels, events are set out as climactic, whereas in *The Good Soldier* they are presented as (Dowell's) afterthoughts. For instance, Dowell frequently forgets things, leaving us in the dark. Confessing, from first base, an ignorance of things, this motivated forgetting shields him from distasteful, threatening, information. So, unaware of the massive denial that underpins it, he insists that all is darkness, one can know nothing with certainty. But this doesn't mean that he lacks feeling: actually, unlike the others, he behaves throughout with some degree of ethics. True, he has been complicit in his own deception but what the eye doesn't see can be strangely comforting and even when he 'opens his eyes', this doesn't lead to greater clarity. Like the people chained up in Plato's Cave (Plato, 2003) they come to believe that the flickering shadows on a wall in front of them are real. Unable to move they don't realise that these are actually reflections of plants and animals that walk behind them but in front of a huge fire. Socrates (Plato's mouthpiece) asks if it's reasonable for these people to take the shadows as the 'real thing', the infrastructure of their society. When one of them escapes he continues to be unable to name the objects causing the shadows and still takes them as real. If compelled to look at the fire he will go blind. If forced into an understanding he may become angry and resist interpretation all the more. As with any allegory, it can represent a great deal but essentially this one examines what governs human perception. Its age-old theme of resistance to change is well borne out as are, as well, the comforts we find in sameness. But more so do stratagems of denial arise if forced to look at the flame (of knowledge) the possibility of 'getting burned' makes us look away.

As a novel *The Good Soldier* is like a hall of mirrors, so constructed that, whilst one is always looking straight at a perfectly solid surface, one is made

to contemplate not the bright surface itself, but the bewildering maze of past circumstances and future consequence that – somewhat falsely – it contains.
(Schorer, 1995: 306)

Psychoanalytically, past, present and future are, at the same time, present. We are never 'here and now' and to believe that we are is mistaken. Ford's story is the unravelling of an unconscious: 'within this text', says Haslam (2002: 57), 'Ford pays attention, employing delaying tactics, to the nature of his characters as they perform, ignore, are jealous and frantic about, repress, sex.' Thus we can conceive of Dowell as a psychotherapist facing resistance, 'his' characters unwilling/unable to disclose that which is hidden to them. Matters emerge grudgingly and – consistent with Heider's theory – psychologically deceitfully. Psychoanalysis confronts fabrication because unlike other therapies it knows that people possess only part knowledge of themselves and of others.

Thus, in Act I, sc vii, do the Macbeths steal into each other's sub-consciousness. Through projective identification (PI) they unify monstrousness, over and over playing off one another, sides of the same coin until they seem as one psyche:

Macbeth:
Prithee, peace,
I dare do all that may become a man:
Who dares do more is none.

Lady Macbeth:
What beast was't, then,
That made you break this enterprise to me?
When you durst do it, then you were a man.

When she tells him that, though a woman, she would kill an infant had she so promised *him*, the inference is clear: destroying her sex she reconstitutes it as male venom, projecting it into his milky heart. Despising her for this, yet does he acquiesce, exclaiming:

Bring forth men-children only!
For thy undaunted mettle should compose
Nothing but males.

Melodrama is avoided by Macbeth's retention of irony, his annoying capacity to see the fallout from different sides. He needs constant telling to 'put a brave face on things', to mock the time with show, to sustain civility even at the expense of truth.

Similarly are the four characters in *The Good Soldier* conceived of as interrelated elements, as chamber music, and to the same purpose; a unity greater than the sum of its parts. Both the Ashburnhams and the Dowells are 'civilised society', the manifestations of this, their large roomy houses, the presence of listening servants, the social etiquette that makes the Ashburnham's thirteen years of silence plausible. Architecture – as we know from the asylums – organises conversation, the high-walled chambers of the big houses easy spaces to escape into. These are people, wrapped in dirty linen, the imperative of whose class is never to be seen washing it in public. In Alan Bennett's *An Englishman Abroad* (1983) an upper-class English traitor, Guy Burgess, living in post-Stalinist Russia, befriends a touring theatre company. Its leading lady promises to send him some items from England which he still craves. In a post-Thatcher meritocratic Britain she tries to buy Burgess some handmade shoes in a shop recently taken over by an aspiring arriviste. Recognising the shoe fit as Burgess's he rejects the purchase with jingoist venom. Handmade ties are next and again recognition ensues. This time however 'the old school' have retained ownership of the shop. With knowing looks of recognition the actress murmurs: 'mum's the word eh?' to which the shopkeeper replies: 'mum is *always* the word'.

What about me?

But what of the person(s) involved, the 'me' element, what Carl Rogers supposed was a 'self', capable of choosing, of moving on? His mantra 'on becoming a person' implied an abstract personhood to which all could attain 'self-actualisation'. The idea is that living successfully is about deciding to grow and become congruent with the world. It's certainly a wholesome way of looking at things although it leaves aside the nastier sides of people as history shows.

The Dowells and the Ashburhams give the lie to Rogerianism in that for them actualisation always entails making sense of others' duplicity, duplicities that stem from unconscious, survivalist, impulses, the avoidance of *thanatos*. When, therefore, their social interactions fail to comfort, anxiety begins to make itself felt. Is it surprising that, for Dowell, 'the breaking up of our little four square coterie was … an unthinkable event?' (pp. 11–12). Not really if seen as the genesis of personal (not just and social) destruction? From this we infer that Dowell's emasculation comes through psychological engagement with others. Things happen *in relation* and the boundaries – remember Macbeth and the witches? – are porous especially when great events are in the offing. And, once begun, if matters fall apart, then one makes wilder choices as a way of reconfiguring things. In *The Good Soldier* four people are stranded at the end of an epoch-shattering war (Chapter 3) bereft of the class-based certainties that preceded it. Likening their relationships to a minuet harks back to when social confidence and its attendant frivolities had their place. Now the lights are fading fast, their decaying lifestyle betokening denial and resistance. Each one plays on the falsehoods of the others, their perceptions of each other's motives, secondary reflections of deceit. Truth becomes an exchange commodity.

But what, this novel wants to know, *is* truth? What is meant when Dowell reminisces that their minuet was in fact a prison packed with hysterics? Wasn't the sunshine real enough, the water in the fountains wet and the music sweet? And, he reflects, if that's what we four were, as we sat and listened, warming in the sun – pretending or otherwise – wasn't that still the truth of what was happening? One thinks again of Goffman's (1990) theories about role and its governance of interactions, how we present our 'selves' to others, or Garfinkel's (1967) students constructing 'realities' from chance. Nothing seems to be what is, except what we make it. Old Mr Hurlbird (p. 20) dies at eighty-four, leaving his extraordinary heart to science, only we discover there's nothing wrong with his heart, just enough symptoms to convince everyone that there was. Perhaps truth lies in appearances? Dowell has lived his life by this principle: self-deceived, he has been constrained by a repression energised by the complicity of others. When eventually he must face the realities of adultery and dishonesty so as to square these with his faith in appearances, he can't do it. No more perhaps than any of us. Might marriages of convenience, for instance, were they to achieve a modicum of success, be any the less real than an arrangement freely entered into? And would not such a marriage merit the soubriquet 'good'? What *are* the demarcations of 'good', 'healthy' relationships anyway? Must there be absolute truth, if such were possible, or do relationships gain some endurance via duplicity and the comforts which it brings?

Shuttlecock

In *Jake's Thing* (this volume, Chapter 4) Jake placates his wife's accusations by accepting and responding to their face value whilst submerging and retaining his true feelings and beliefs. What does this leave his wife, Brenda, to go on? How do we know that what Jake tells her is in any sense true? The fact is we don't know, any more than we do generally. Always we face the problem of how to interpret communication in this or that context.

In *Not Made of Wood* (1974) Jan Foudraine introduces a patient diagnosed as having nihilistic delusions. The patient constantly states that he is 'not made of wood' but is ignored given psychiatry's concern with the form of delusions, not their intrinsic content. Foudraine says that the patient really means: 'I have feelings', 'I am not solid', 'please listen to me'. Of the same generation as R.D. Laing, Foudraine was interested in the symbolism of psychotic speech, believing that language gave off signs of therapeutic usefulness. So that when, in *The Good Soldier,* Nancy Rufford, in her madness, utters 'shuttlecock' repeatedly we recognise that she has been pushed this way and that, from pillar to post, between Edward and Leonora. More so however does 'shuttlecock' signify that all of us are battered by fate and circumstance as well as the difficulty of gauging some truth from what is said to us. In Discussion Ten (p. 218–21) a concept of projective identification is argued to be an important process by which we acquire understanding of why people behave as they do. In everyday life we may have to forego this so that our lives may come to resemble that of the Ashburnhams and the Dowells. As therapists, however, we need to avoid the risky business of taking people at their word.

Film

The Cave is an animated adaptation of Plato's famous allegory and was produced in 2008. Written and directed by Michael Ramsey it was produced by Bullhead Entertainment based in Thornton, Colorado. It has won numerous awards all over the world and might be an excellent introduction into what is an enlightening but still challenging metaphor.

References

Amis, K (1992) *Memoirs*. London: Penguin Books.

Armstrong, PB (1987) *The Challenge of Bewilderment*. London: Cornell University Press.

Bennett, A (1983) *An Englishman Abroad*. BBC Television Drama, 29 November.

Ford, FM (1995) *The Good Soldier*. London: W.W. Norton & Co. (Original work published 1915)

Foudraine, J (1974) *Not Made of Wood*. London: Quartet Books.

Garfinkel, H (1967) *Studies in Ethnomethodology*. New Jersey: Prentice-Hall.

Goffman, E (1990) *The Presentation of Self in Everyday Life*. London: Penguin.

Haslam, S (2002) *Fragmenting Modernism*. Manchester: Manchester University Press.

Heider, F (1958) *The Psychology of Interpersonal Relations*. New York: Wiley.

Hynes, S (1995) The epistemology of 'The Good Soldier'. In M Stannard (ed) *The Good Soldier* (pp 310–17). London: W.W. Norton & Co.

Levenson, M (2004) *Modernism and the Fate of Individuality*. Cambridge: Cambridge University Press.

Meixner, JA (1962) *Ford Madox Ford's Novels: A critical study*. London: Oxford University Press.

Plato (2003) *The Republic*. London: Penguin Classics.

Ramsey, M (2008) *The Cave* [film]. Boulder, CO: Spoken Image Films.

Schorer, M (1995) 'The Good Soldier' as comedy. In M Sannard (ed) *The Good Soldier* (pp 305–10). London: W.W. Norton & Co.

Shakespeare, W (1967) *Macbeth*. Harmondsworth: Penguin.

Smiley, J (2006) The odd couples. *The Guardian,* Saturday, 27 May.

Tóibín, C (2007) Paper addressed to conference: Ford Madox Ford: Visual arts and media. 17–19 September. Genova: Universita degli Studi di Genova.

Trotter, D (2001) *Paranoid Modernism*. Oxford: Oxford University Press.

CONCLUSION

I hope that you enjoyed reading (at least) some of my selection and are propelled further into fiction as a means of understanding mental health and its absence. Of course as I mentioned before, other therapists have interested themselves in make-believe. Professor Jerry Gans (Harvard University) has written enlighteningly about Kafka and it was he who recommended *The Good Soldier* to me in respect of its links with psychoanalytic concepts. Equally, has British psychiatrist Femi Oyebode (2009) engaged with a range of literature within clinical discourse. Some of Oyebode's (2002) favourites include *The Labyrinths* (Borges, 1964), *One Hundred Years of Solitude* (Garcia Márquez, 1967), *The Outsider*, (Camus, 1982) and *Crowds and Power* (Canetti, 1962). Pertinently, he writes (2002: 445) about Canetti that although his 'insights are often false, it is the liveliness of his ideas, the sheer originality of his approach, that makes him immensely readable.' This was the driving force behind my text, to initiate discussion on mental distress that would help shunt psychiatric – including psychotherapeutic – discussion away from reductionism.

Another influence has been psychiatrist David Goldberg (2001) whose choices include *Fathers and Sons* (Turgenev, 1965), *Scarlet and Black* (Stendhal, 1972), *The Rack* (Ellis, 1961), *The Horse's Mouth* (Cary, 1944) and *Myra Breckinridge* (Vidal, 1968). In an interesting passage, he identifies the nineteenth-century novel – I imagine he had women novelists in mind – as prefiguring Brown and Harris's (1978) seminal treatise on female oppression, humiliation, as the genesis of clinical depression. Curiously, Goldberg goes on to say (2001: 88) that: 'the achievement of Brown and Harris has been to take case histories from real life and then to use nomothetic [naming] methods to investigate relationships between depression and social variables. No amount of novel-reading does that!' Possibly not, but what it can do is add importantly to that which *is* named from writing that informs 'the social' creatively and imaginatively. No amount of qualitative investigations matches the energising force of fiction when it enters the heads of its subjects under the enquiring gaze of its readers. Further, nothing outside fiction conveys the effrontery that psychological science can induce in an intelligent person than that conveyed in Amis's *Jake's Thing* (this volume, Chapter 4). Jake's visceral distaste when confronted with the demand to *be* psychological, or, in his case, to be anything, lies on the page like the sticky effusion of a snail. Neither does formal psychology contribute to how madness is understood and played out in relationships. When it tries to, for example in Transactional Analysis (Berne, 1966), it collapses into absurdly wide characterisations of 'the child', 'the adult', or 'the parent' as if such external, abstract, forms exist in any sense not arbitrated by history, economics, ethnicity or culture. Similarly, when it encapsulates the process of interaction as somehow conforming to predetermined scripts it flings open the door to a pop psychology within the reach of 'therapists' enamoured of its suitcase language and fey assumptions.

Why we read

In respect of *why* we read novels (or go to the theatre) the element of enjoyment is not easily dismissed. I have dealt (implicitly) with this in Chapter One in respect of potboilers, comparing them to 'serious' or literary alternatives. Yet particular genres don't prevent us bringing complex attitudinal or analytic attention to them. In this, our concern is not the social psychology of who reads which novels or why, but rather how different kinds of books can enlighten psychological understanding.

Rieger (1994: 27) states that 'literature is a record of those elusive moments at which life is alone fully itself, fulfilled in consciousness and form'. So that whilst fiction is (in itself) not real, it informs us about reality, especially its 'incomplete status' and it can do this since it doesn't carry the promised expectations of psychology research with its hypotheses and anticipated outcomes. Neither does fiction seek to inform didactically, albeit we have discussed the 'factual' as an aspect of the postcolonial novel. Instead it constantly demands collusion from readers in respect of its meanings, construing itself in ways that complicate this requirement endlessly. Thus in Chapter 11 (this volume) are the 'characters displayed as different sides of the same person' or in Chapter 8 (this volume) where we can't rely on the narrator to tell the truth because, in truth, he doesn't know the truth either. It's a salutary lesson that questions what can be known with any finality.

It is to fiction alone that we gain entry to a believable consciousness of others. We must trust the genius of writers that they are giving us reasonable facsimiles of human psychology but we can test this by entering their fiction and I suggest that we become convinced of the likely truth of a writer's vision when the work stays with us indefinably but lingeringly. True, cheap thrillers can be unputdownable but this satiates curiosity about endings only, the 'what happens next' fixation, rarely leaving us troubled or enlightened about our own lives.

As mental health students we appreciate writers who allow us to see the awfulness of dispossession and rejection when experienced from alienation, whether phenomenological or social. Gregor Samsa (this volume, Chapter 7) stands for every schizophrenic who has been awarded the designation 'outsider'. We touched upon this directly but as well within contexts of gender and race where the outsider status stems from collective racial and male chauvinist prejudices. A society needs its outsiders, its 'theys', because if it wasn't for 'they', things would hardly appear to get better. We have, in relation to madness, come a long way from prescriptive rejection, in no small way this comes from the humanities, from valuing individuality and ceasing to regard what persons say as a type of talk, a type of belief, but as something inherently meaningful. This is not to minimise clinical data but to say that it's at its best when cultured by wider considerations of what it is to be human in a sometimes lousy world.

We began by questioning ourselves outside the comfort zone of standard texts that revolve around questions whose fundamental attributes have already been settled. Concepts of first rank symptoms in schizophrenia may invite some intellectual review that skirts around the details of their applicability but this hardly affects how we, as therapists, come closer to the experiences of others. Only by setting aside, even temporarily, the privileged language systems of the learned – Foucault foolishly suggests abandoning rationality itself – can we conjure up space in our own heads and enjoin the languages of fiction. Reading a work of fiction or watching a play is like entering a dream where the usual rules of social engagement don't apply and where we see our fears and anticipations as they can be and not conflated by theory, though let's not disregard the latter. It's just that, in our society, that which empirically 'flies' in any objective, reductive, sense is that which get the kudos and the research monies!

For me, fiction is at its best and most interestingly difficult when it scans the matrices which constitute madness and the reactions it brings about. Whether it be Gregor Samsa, Harry Haller or Jake Richardson, the problem of what to say, how to act and react, is seen as a major human predicament. In *Notes from the Underground* (Dostoevsky, 2006) avoiding totalitarianism means super-imposing on rationality an exercise of free choice. Even when it spells disaster, better to choose and to think hard over one's choice, than to just follow the form or the requirement. This may make you misunderstood and warrant local or universal rejection but, like Felicia and the others, solace is attained in the underground of the streets, from having held out against the madness of conformity.

References

Berne, E (1966) *Games People Play*. London: Andre Deutsch.

Borges, JL (1964) *The Labyrinths*. New York: New Directions.

Brown, GW & Harris, T (1978) *The Social Origins of Depression*. London: Tavistock.

Camus, A (1982) *The Outsider*. London: Hamish Hamilton.

Canetti, E (1962) *Crowds and Power*. London: Gollancz.

Cary, J (1944) *The Horse's Mouth*. London: Michael Joseph.

Dostoevsky, F (2006) *Notes from the Underground*. London: Hesperus.

Ellis, AE (1961) *The Rack*. Harmondsworth: Penguin.

Goldberg, D (2001) Ten books. *British Journal of Psychiatry. 178,* 88–91.

Garcia Márquez, G (1967) *One Hundred Years of Solitude.* London: Harper & Row.

Oyebode, F (2002) Ten books. *British Journal of Psychiatry, 181,* 445–9.

Oyebode, F (2009) *Mindreadings: Literature and psychiatry.* London: Royal College of Psychiatrists.

Rieger, BM (1994) *Dionysus in Literature.* Bowling Green, OH: State University Popular Press.

Stendhal (1953) *Scarlet and Black.* Harmondsworth: Penguin.

Turgenev, I (1965) *Fathers and Sons.* Harmondsworth: Penguin.

Vidal, G (1968) *Myra Breckinridge.* London: Anthony Blond.

DISCUSSION ONE

Chapter Two: *Fiction and Madness*

R.D. Laing

To say that R.D. Laing was psychiatry's greatest star is no exaggeration, albeit a star whose radiance faded fast. In that most radical of periods, the 1960s, he was the most prominent of a group of theoretical agitators identified as anti-psychiatrists. Not only did he acquire a dissident status within his profession, he was also lauded on TV, the college speakers' circuit and with rear car window stickers proclaiming 'I'm crazy about R.D. Laing'.

As a medical student, Laing acquired an interest in existential philosophy. Upon qualifying, he naturally gravitated towards psychiatry yet with serious reservations about some of its practices. As a young doctor in Glasgow's Gartnavel Hospital, he befriended some women patients who had become institutionalised in a 'back ward' and he allowed them to befriend him. He renamed this ward 'the rumpus room' which gives some indication of what it was like. As the late professor of psychiatry, Anthony Clare, put it: 'Laing put the person back into psychiatry'; in fact Laingian ideas had persuaded Clare to become a psychiatrist. In this, he was referring to Laing's first (and most important) book *The Divided Self* (1960) and although Laing would write prolifically, this remains his most cogent work on schizophrenia.

Unlike Szasz in *The Myth of Mental Illness* (1961/1976) Laing never denied the existence of schizophrenia but rather explained it in a radically different way. His premises were:

1. Psychiatrists pay insufficient (if any) attention to the experiences of schizophrenics.
2. How the 'illness' is experienced is crucial to its understanding.
3. The social matrix of 'the patient', especially his family, is important to understanding the 'condition'.
4. The 'schizophrenic' is an 'elected victim' whose role is to act out a madness that properly resides in the family.
5. Treatment lies not in drugs or physical treatments but in coming to terms with this 'illness' experientially and socially.
6. Essentially, schizophrenia is a sane reaction to a potential or actual threatening world, as sane as any other of response.
7. It is, in fact, 'another way of being human'.

This created a stir at the time because it diametrically opposed Karl Jaspers' (1883–1969) highly influential theory that psychiatrists should diagnose symptoms, that the form of hallucinations and delusions should take precedence over their content (1913/1997). Of course in the 1960s, provocative, modish-sounding, daring, revolutionary ideas were par for the course. But that this reflected authentic shifts in cultural norms or was merely decorative, socially skin deep, remains debatable. The fact is, Laing's ideas were not adopted by orthodox psychiatry even if he drew attention to the dehumanising aspects of, especially, hospital practice. His further claims about the detrimental effects of families on the genesis of schizophrenia made a small dent in medical circles. Conceptually this was his most daring insult (to formal psychiatry), his contention that families selectively induce schizophrenia in their young, that an adolescent family member – the elected victim – inhabits a madness that is familial in origin.

But first there was Ronny's stardom, even notoriety, and boy did he enjoy it! He allowed himself all the adulation that sixties' audiences were so willing to give him. His guru status was particularly reinforced on college campuses by those who gasped for the oxygen of dissent. The resultant deterioration of his work, the failure to develop ideas led to a slow drift into showmanship, regaling audiences with ever more wild pronouncements (often slurred) on the nature of madness. In *The Politics of Experience and the Bird of Paradise* (Laing, 1967) he seemed to say that schizophrenia was a mystical journey towards higher levels of insight to which the 'sane' were denied access. He wrote poetry, recorded an LP, appeared on television, not always sober, and generally entertained audiences with his 'presence' and clever articulation. But the drift into mysticism was a step too far and in any event the times were catching up with radicalism. In many ways the sixties were invented in the seventies and what's most remarkable, with hindsight, is the very great number of those, professionals or otherwise, who were not remotely affected by it.

Laing so wanted to write another substantial book but it wasn't to be, although there is always in his writings material both entertaining and challenging. Like his psychiatrist colleague, David Cooper, he was wrecked by alcohol, although he stopped drinking a year before he died. By then he had dropped out of sight although he could joke about this: 'A woman came up to me the other day and said, "did you used to be R.D. Laing?"' One still hears his name bandied about in psychiatric circles (Reed, 2009) but any regeneration of his ideas is a forlorn hope in a climate that worships evidence, measured outcomes and conformity.

In respect of families and schizophrenia, he would always deny that he had said that conflicted families *cause* schizophrenia, that what he had actually said was that schizophrenia is an intelligible reaction to situations of intense family stress. However, the dividing line is narrow here and he did wait a very long time to absolve himself from the original criticism. Curiously, later empirical studies (Leff et al, 1982) did confirm that family interactions can affect the illness pathways of patients, that patients subjected to negative, critical, emotion deteriorate whereas those in more nurturing environments improve. However, the distinction between causation and exacerbation is crucial and Laing made a mistake when he inferred causation.

What always seemed dubious was how or why one young member of a family became its 'elected victim'. In their book *Sanity, Madness and the Family* (Laing & Esterson, 1964) all of the patients are adolescent, all operate within families whose parental elements are belligerent and destructive. But why, where there are several siblings, does one become ill and not another? Perhaps the relevant factor might be gender or it might be age, the problem being that any concept of 'elected victim' supposes collusion, the victim putting himself forward. Laing was a psychoanalyst and I imagine that something like projective identification (this volume, Chapter 11) played a part in how he perceived schizophrenic behaviour, how he formulated his family thesis. So that when one of the family, unable to contain fear and anger, projects this into his family where it is taken up and used against him, and as he tries to deal with this by splitting from consciousness the cycle continues to a point where his conflicted behaviour proceeds towards victimhood.

Laing's contribution lay in his cutting a swathe through a moribund, medicalised, psychiatry. That he was wrong in some of the detail doesn't detract from the vigour he brought to acknowledging patients for who they are. What he provided was an intellectual enquiry into what 'the schizophrenic' was feeling and thinking and with the aim of making professional responses to this palpably human. His failure was in subsuming the humanity imperative beneath an ill-worked-through philosophy that enhanced his reputation (amongst some) but was of little practical utility.

References

Jaspers, K (1997) *General Psychopathology*. London: Johns Hopkins University Press. (Original work published 1913)

Laing, RD (1960) *The Divided Self*. London: Tavistock.

Laing, RD (1967) *The Politics of Experience and the Bird of Paradise*. Harmondsworth: Penguin.

Laing, RD & Esterson, A (1964) *Sanity, Madness and the Family*. London: Tavistock.

Leff, J, Kuipers, L & Berkowitz, T (1982) A controlled trial of social intervention in the families of schizophrenic patients. *British Journal of Psychiatry, 141*, 121–34.

Reed, A (2009) Revisiting RD Laing. *Mental Health Practice, 12* (6), 16–19.

Szasz, T (1976) *The Myth of Mental Illness,* 2nd ed. New York: Harper and Row.

DISCUSSION TWO

Chapter 12: *A Question of Power*

The postcolonial novel and writing back

Marxist theoretician Antonio Gramsci (1891–1937) said that to exploit a nation you had, necessarily, to impose cultural supremacy over it. Guns and prisons played their part, but inculcating belief in the ascendant status of the colonising force was *the* prerequisite, the subjected group becoming 'the other', rewritten into history, literature and art as inferior. The term 'writing back' (Ashcroft et al, 2002) denotes fiction written from the vantage point of previously colonised groups and which, within their narratives, engages with colonialism and its effects in political and economic terms. Thus a postcolonial novel like *A Question of Power* (Chapter 12) affirms the mores and concerns of an indigenous group against white racism and it is this that makes it a force in African literature. More particularly, Head writes back to protest the effects of colonisation on people's mental health. Reflecting on the 'merits' of Western teaching and African history, Elizabeth, Head's protagonist, (Head, 1974: 134) says:

> There's some such thing as black people's suffering being a summary of everything the philosophers and prophets ever said. They said, never think along lines of I and mine. It is death. Black people learned that lesson brutally because they were the living victims of the greed inspired by I and mine.

One of my observations, as a teacher, has been the difficulty that some overseas students have with our Western attachment to 'I' and the 'self'. It's a difficulty that conceivably stems from intuitive distrust of self-aggrandisement in whatever terms. It's a small observation but its miniature standing doesn't detract from our obligation to explore the implications of ethnic cultures in relation to therapeutic practice.

Difference

The postcolonial novel's importance is that it merges autobiography with politics and economics to show how these negatively impact on its characters. Of course all fiction writers utilise experience, that's not an issue. However, in the postcolonial novel there can occur an intrusion of persons and events so arbitrarily that you are left wondering if it's a novel at all. And the issue is not the kinds of intrusions where problems, within the story, interplay with the novelist's identity or with literary theory. Rather are postcolonial intrusions factual, taking the form of political tracts, even *speeches,* which don't arise organically from the narrative. Quick to pounce, Western critics begrudged African novels much significance beyond the parochial, seeing them driven as much by political ideology as by literary creativity. As Achebe (1975: 3) bitterly observed: 'The latter day colonialist critic ... given to big-brother arrogance, sees the African writer as a somewhat unfinished European who with patient guidance will grow up one day and write like every other European.'

For Achebe (1975) it's asking the impossible for African writers to forego rage against racism and corruption and, to the extent that they won't, they suffer for 'their art' not only from Eng. Lit. critics, but from African despots as well. Not unusually, African novelists go to gaol. Head's novel rages more than most, wrapping anger with madness and gender, it uniquely describes the political as predisposing mental breakdown. This is a dense, somewhat didactic, fiction, a narrative bereft of psychiatric simplicity or literary niceties; it barks but rightfully so.

As Jameson (1986: 69) notes:

> Third world texts, even those which are seemingly private and invested with properly libidinal dynamic necessarily project a political dimension in the form of national allegory: the story of the private individual destiny always an allegory of the embattled situation of the public third world culture and society.

However, we may still ask *how* literature informs us about nations? In Head's case this would mean reading her novel as history and this would be difficult since novels invite multiple interpretations. This is not so with history which seeks some continuity with beliefs, actual events and facts. In essence the question turns on whether the personal can be political or indeed can ever not be political. There is much in Elizabeth's character that echoes South African racial oppression but problems arise when fictional characters become conduits for political arguments about this. This doesn't happen too much in Head's novel because Elizabeth is grounded in psychological distress with the politics and race, albeit deeply felt, forming a provocative background

Variants

Vestiges of writing back continue amongst women writers even when living in England: black novelists like Zadie Smith (*White Teeth,* 2000) and Andrea Levy (*Small Island,* 2004) assess questions of migration, race and multiculturalism:

Rejecting where necessary the language and forms of those who once colonised them, or appropriating, manipulating or subverting that language and those forms to their own end.

(Padley, 2006: 73)

You might also consider to what extent the description of the postcolonial or write-back novel can be attached to William Trevor's *Felicia's Journey* (this volume, Chapter 8), a story whose undercurrents of relationships between Ireland and England are played out as comparisons between innocence, on the one hand, and psychopathic malevolence on the other.

Finally, observe the absence of black people in the nineteenth-century novels of the Imperial period. Which is not to say their presence is unfelt. The Creole or mixed-race undercurrents of madness in *Jane Eyre*, for instance, testify to the lineage behind Head's *A Question of Power* and to the generalised idea of madness as a blood degeneration of sorts.

References

Achebe, C (1975) *Morning Yet on Creation Day*. London: Heinemann.
Ashcroft, B, Griffith, G & Tiffen, H (2002) *The Empire Writes Back*. London: Routledge.
Head, B (1974) *A Question of Power*. London: Heinemann.
Levy, A (2004) *Small Island*. London: Review Books.
Jameson, F (1986) Third world literature in the era of multinational capitalism. *Social Text* XV, 65–88.
Padley, S (2006) *Key Concepts in Contemporary Literature*. Basingstoke: Palgrave.
Smith, Z (2000) *White Teeth*. London: Hamish Hamilton.

DISCUSSION THREE
Chapter 7: *Metamorphosis*

Erving Goffman

The most influential sociologist of his generation, Goffman contributed significantly to psychiatry mainly through his book *Asylums* (1961/1968). A scintillating text, it quickly became a reference point for the activities of anti-psychiatric practitioners, theorists and researchers. Although unhappy with the term 'Symbolic Interactionism', this is usually designated as Goffman's main conceptual starting point. In essence it contains three basic assumptions: that we act towards people and events through the meanings we assign to them; that these meanings will stem from social interactions; and that interpretation will alter or reorganise these meanings via who and how we encounter events.

In effect, individuals work their way in and about a given society by interpreting the signs contained in language or action. Some elements of interaction may be interpreted as powerful and/or influential, their demands difficult to resist, in many cases needing to be assuaged. Part of how we cope with disproportionately powerful people is to present ourselves differently within the forms and structures that we share with them. Goffman (1959/1990) called such interpersonal manoeuvrings the 'presentation of self in everyday life'. It's as though we are in a continually unfolding drama – of which we are not the author – where we are called upon to perform in response to who we meet and in what context. We may be extremely adept at this and as one politician once acutely remarked: 'the way to get along is to go along'. We could do worse than reflect upon the latter in respect of our occupational, parental or other aspirational lives.

Goffman's work is relevant to mental health in that he showed how social mores punish those deemed to be deviating from these. In chapter one of *Asylums*, 'On the Characteristics of Total Institutions', he introduced the idea of 'social stripping', which was soon in use to describe the admission procedures of mental hospitals as transformations designed to eliminate the everyday indices of personhood. Unsurprisingly, the American National Institute for Mental Health dissuaded Goffman from publishing the book. A wise move on their part for although *Asylums* didn't sound the death knell of institutionalisation it delivered a body blow to its more blatant features.

Goffman was a good writer and, what's more, his book was based on actual observations and so therefore influential in pushing forward qualitative research with its emphasis on assessing persons within social systems. *Asylums* was less about psychiatry per se but arriving at the same time as Thomas Szasz's *The Myth of Mental Illness* (1961) and Laing's *The Divided Self* (1960) it helped substantiate a powerful critique of conventional psychiatric practices. From Goffman, we derive such concepts as 'Total Institution' with its regimentalism and detrimental effects on all who are subject to their rules. We also get the word *stigma* which immediately attached itself to the critical reactions which mentally ill people often face. Soon, he will define deviance, not as a sign of derision, but as a socially constructed index of threats that attend anyone who stands apart from supposed norms.

The deviance angle freed radical psychiatrists from established medical nostrums enabling them to envisage the schizophrenic as 'outsider', living on the edges of society, a veritable non-conformist. This meant that they could ascribe to psychotic people the same capacity to socially construct their worlds, to see them as interpreting matters as they saw them, through interaction, and especially in family terms. In effect, all of us present a self differently whether defensively, aggressively or metaphorically. We all possess instincts or desires and wants that reflect passing fancies. We are forever in a constant, changing, process of being all things to all people.

Of course, you may think that little of this is new (this volume, Chapter 7) and as Shakespeare noted some few hundred years ago:

> All the world's a stage.
> And all the men and women merely players:
> They have their exists and their entrances;
> And one man in his time plays many parts,
> His acts being seven ages.
>   (*As You Like It,* Act II, sc vii)

Nor is the Bard unaware of the interpretive mountains to be climbed as we apply meanings to utterances whose psychological origins we may only guess. Listen (*Macbeth*, Act V, sc v) as Lady Macbeth whispers in her husband's ear:

> To beguile the time,
> Look like the time; bear welcome in your eye,
> Your hand, your tongue: look like the innocent flower,
> But be the serpent under't.

For Shakespeare, the cosmos and its particular deviances bring about a strange complicity, infected emotion runs amok and once let loose becomes hard to stop it up again.

> To-morrow, and to-morrow, and to-morrow
> Creeps in this petty pace from day to day,

To the last syllable of recorded time;
And all our yesterdays have lighted fools
The way to dusty death.
    (*Macbeth*, Act V, sc v)

True, and spoken by someone at the end of his tether. But its inevitableness touches us all as does its pessimism in respect of human autonomy. Goffman systematised ideas of individuals being acted on in society. He believed that society came first in that one could not subject it to a capricious free will that otherwise circumvents its 'effects' and one can see in this, that in the whole representing more than its parts, there lies a truth of sorts.

References

Goffman, E (1968) *Asylums*. Harmondsworth: Penguin Books. [Original work published 1961]

Goffman, E (1990) *The Presentation of Self in Everyday Life*. Harmondsworth: Penguin. [Original work published 1959]

Laing, RD (1960) *The Divided Self*. London: Tavistock.

Shakespeare, W (1967) *Macbeth*. Harmondsworth: Penguin.

Shakespeare, W (1968) *As You Like It*. Harmondsworth: Penguin.

Szasz, T (1961) *The Myth of Mental Illness*. New York: Harper and Row. (2nd ed, 1976)

DISCUSSION FOUR

Chapter 3: *Regeneration*

Freud

So much can be said about for and against him that it's difficult to know where to start. Best to stick with the main tenets of his work – for a comprehensive account of his life and work see Gay (1989), which is readable and informative. Also, any short summary of his ideas will inevitably gloss over sometimes complex, even contradictory-seeming, propositions. That said, I will try to cover the main points of his theory and practice as palatably as I can.

Dr Sigmund Freud (1856–1939) was a physician practising and writing in Vienna until 1938 when he came to London to escape the Nazis. His work may be taken as both a philosophy of life and as a way of doing therapy called Psychoanalysis. His approach, also sometimes called psychodynamic or depth psychology, posits an unconscious mind impacting on manifest (behavioural) decisions, actions and speech. This unconscious domain is comprised of motivations and conflicts that are difficult to discern via ordinary discourse, requiring instead a lengthy analysis using Freudian techniques.

True to his time (and training) Freud saw life in scientific terms. His was a perspective that prized cause and effect, mechanics, explanation rather than description or opinion. Unsurprisingly therefore he contended that behaviour was not an end point in itself but needed a cause, a system of determinants by which it could be explained or even predicted. These determinants coalesced in early childhood with the onset of conflicts occurring at important developmental stages. For instance, the often difficult manner by which children acquire the social rudiments involved in defecation (potty training) can become a focus from which problematic, for instance obsessive, behaviour emerges in adult life. So too is the development of sexual identity, a journey fraught with issues of the identity of self and others as one attains a mature sexual status. The means by which these conflicts become unconscious is called repression (not to be confused with the conscious activity of suppression), one of a group of mental mechanisms or, preferably, defensive processes that are themselves not wholly conscious. Repression works like this: painful emotions that result from clashes between desire and reality are pushed into unconsciousness where, however, they remain active, surfacing during dreams or as anxiety or other dysfunctional states. Indeed consciousness can be seen as a tapestry of these mechanisms as they work deceptively to sustain themselves whilst granting us the illusion of conscious determinism. For instance, one acquires a store of anger from particular encounters but which is displaced onto another object or person because directing it at an appropriate recipient would be just too dangerous. My boss gives me a hard time but I need my job and his favour: so my rage is redirected towards my wife albeit without realising the shift involved. Or recall Basil Fawlty, enraged at a car that won't start, breaking a branch from a tree to beat it into subservience! There are quite a few of these mechanisms and their defensive interplay constitutes what we mistakenly conceive as 'us', the 'me' that ploughs on from one day to the next. If you are perturbed at the paradoxical nature of this – for example the question of what constitutes an unthought thought – you are not alone. But if you reflect on your intolerance of alcoholics, without accessing the memory of your alcoholic father, you may concede the relative truth of motivated or conflicted forgetting.

Time's theories

True to the' hydraulic thinking' of the late nineteenth century, Freud saw the brain as a assembly of compartments realised as Ego, Superego and Id with these corresponding to the conscious, conscience and unconscious respectively. So there is (a) a self, the bit we think we are at any one time; (b) a component (superego) that knows the self but also has 'knowledge' of the unconscious; and (c) the unconscious itself. In spatial terms the self component is an A4-sized sheet of paper, the conscience about quadruple this and the unconscious an area of a thousand football pitches.

So, the unconscious is vast, stuffed with repressed shame and rage that constantly seeks ways of pushing into consciousness. One of its aspects is that it disowns time, everything is at the same time present. Neither does it take account of gender or ethics; indeed the unconscious is best described as a cauldron of boiling liquid about to spill over. Several points of therapeutic interest flow from this. The relevance of the 'here and now' is denied, the notion of growth directed, choices seen as denial, avoiding deeper issues. Instead, the dictum: 'Give me the child until he is seven, and I will show you the man' is paramount with adult problems conceived of as unresolved traumas from childhood. Thus a crucial part of psychoanalytic therapy, its very rationale, is the patient's displacement within therapy of unresolved problems and where the therapist's job is to unravel these by making explicit the whys and wherefores of their unconscious status. The displacement, during therapy, is called 'the transference' and part of Freud's genius in formulating it is that when a patient fell in love with one of his colleagues (a married man who ran a mile from the possible outcomes of this) Freud recognised that the 'love' (or attachment) properly belonged elsewhere and that the therapist/recipient was a constructed medium by which the projected conflict might be held and perhaps dissipated.

The superego watches the cauldron as it boils, keeping it just short of tipping over. It judges certain actions not feasible whether in moral or consequential terms. These are actions which, if ignored, would induce anxiety or other mental distress. But if, by whatever means, repressed material does seep from the unconscious, it will attach itself phobic-like to something incongruous like dirt or spiders, or as an unattached, free-floating, fear that knows no bounds. In a sense the superego keeps the ego in reasonable moral union with society, its precepts and demands.

The practice of psychoanalysis

We can divide this into psychoanalysis proper and psychoanalysis approach. The former requires a commitment on the part of the patient (psychoanalysis retains the term patient) to four or five sessions per week for five years. This is some commitment both in terms of psychic energy but, as well, financially – the pressures on one's family or social life becoming immeasurable. Classically, the Freudian patient lies supine on the proverbial couch while the analyst, sitting slightly behind and out of sight, waits for the session to proceed towards its fifty minute end. The strict adherence to time – the 'golden hour' – is designed to combat the unconscious's recognition of this period. The paradox here is that the patient will begin to divulge important material as the session nears its end; it can, in effect, cheat by seeming to become enlivened. Think of the times you have been 'in group' when it begins to liven up near the finish! It's kind of like two worlds playing cat and mouse with each other with no guarantees on either side. To allow the session to go beyond its allotted time would be to concede too much to the unconscious.

Psychoanalysis approach is when a therapist uses psychoanalytic principles as a means of getting behind what a client says, discerning anxieties that may lie behind statements or behaviour, such as a client lingering by a door when a session has ended. In these cases it would constitute a therapist's eclectic position as one of a series of possible tactics and consonant with a given client's needs. It accepts the idea of an unconscious at play but without wanting to engage in the more arcane practices or at a similar depth as psychoanalysis proper.

As Joel Kovel (1978) says, psychoanalysis is a 'know thyself' therapy that requires knowledge of one's bad bits as well as the good. It's not hard to see how it lost out to the 'here and now' therapies with their 'everybody can be good if they try' standpoint. With psychoanalysis, there comes a point where the human must burn, where the repressed wish is brought into the actual world – albeit initially in the unusual setting of a therapeutic encounter, a boundary between enquiry and living. I referred earlier to defensive processes rather than mechanisms which tend to be depicted in black and white terms. So too the received wisdom that behaviour is driven by an unconscious, which is another misnomer. More accurately, do matters turn on the boundaries of what is imperceptible to both domains and the fear that these perceptions elicit if ever the balance tilts in favour of the repressed.

Freud believed that people would go to any lengths to avoid contact with the psyche and that that included engaging with therapies that *seemed* to do this. Thus the efficiency of cognitive behaviour therapy with a 'condition' like obsessive compulsive disorder (OCD) where the 'symptoms' are quickly eliminated as opposed to psychoanalysis which has never successfully 'treated' it. You might think that with its symbolic grounding and ritually significant behaviours (hand washing, counting etc) OCD was made with psychoanalysis in mind but not so.

Yet what transpires, I think, is that when depth psychology is brought into play with something like OCD, there occurs a 'recognition' that the very root of the problem may be disturbed, thus the immediate and resolute resistance to its advance. This is not to advocate dynamic therapy where it doesn't work but to point out that this particular failure doesn't mean it's untrue.

References

Gay, P (1989) *Freud: A life for our time*. London: Papermac.
Kovel, J (1978) *A Complete Guide to Therapy*. Harmondsworth: Penguin.

DISCUSSION FIVE

Chapter 3: *Regeneration*

What was neurasthenia?

It was the chronic fatigue syndrome of its time. The background to its use as a diagnosis was that late nineteenth century physicians believed that fixed amounts of genetically determined nervous energy circulated the body as a message deliverer. When excessive demands were made on this supply – by too much work, worry or lack of rest, it lost capacity to feed sufficient amounts through to other organs, for example the reproductive system, and neurasthenia kicked in.

This is not as far-fetched as it sounds. At the time, excessive demands on people were fuelled by galloping industrialisation and the urban dehumanisation that flowed from this. Forfeited tranquillity, excessive working hours and corporate requirement induced what we nowadays call 'stress', as nebulous a term as neurasthenia ever was! Clinicians had identified such things as newspapers, steam power, the telegraph, and the sciences generally, as causative factors. In addition there were issues of identity with mass immigration to America producing uncertainties about what it was that actually constituted being American.

As well as this, it was rationalised that whatever the male capacity to withstand pressure, women were far more vulnerable. In fact, the increasing mental activity of women, with growing numbers of them entering college or the professions, with consequent deepening of thought and intellectual challenge, risked depleting their vital energy, not to mention femininity. It is important to understand that this made sense since it was a given that men were more intelligent than women. This being so, women had to try much harder, the problem being that if they did, this simply depleted their energy all the more! Like the men in the trenches, women were constrained by social position and especially the male reasoning that, on one hand, purported to be chivalrous towards them but which attitude defined them as secondary and in need of male support.

Shorter (1997) says that neurasthenia was the prototype for subsequent functional disorders like schizophrenia inasmuch as although you cannot observe its pathology under a microscope it is nevertheless present. I have written elsewhere (Clarke, 1999) about how psychiatric developments acquire enhanced standing through association with (a) a charismatic leader, usually male, but also (b) the production of a book so as to provide intellectual endorsement for the new departure. So when S. Weir Mitchell wrote *Fat and Blood* (1878), neurasthenia took off as a disorder of widespread application. Comprising symptoms of insomnia, depression, fatigue, muscle pain, indigestion, headaches, lack of concentration and anxiety meant that it could be applied to all and sundry. Then as now, the psychopharmacological industry sprang to the fore offering its wares as an instant and effective solution. By this time, in the US, the condition had become so prevalent amongst the well-to-do that it was being called Americanitis. Without more ado, an Americanitis Elixir arrived on the market at 75 cents a bottle, no doubt benefiting those who believed in it.

Barker's novel

In *Regeneration*, neurasthenia is the catalyst that conjoins illness as a social construction to events in civilian and military life. By the book's end, we come face to face with an insane war that immerses human beings in faecal and blood-drenched trenches. Whilst the generals execute those who cannot stand it any more, they do little to halt the slaughter. That they executed those not of their own kind underscores neurasthenia as a disorder with class parameters. This was an illness that attracted the upper classes like flies to fly-paper such that everyone in the novel, doctors and patients alike, end up twitching or stammering. Halfway through, Dr Rivers states: 'I already stammer and I'm starting to twitch' (1992: 140).

It's the war that is driving everyone insane; the war is the real illness and there is nothing any of them can do about it. The trenches are more than dugouts in the mud, they are a devastating compound of expectations and restrictions the soldiers must face with only recourse to death or the small chance of insanity. It was the waiting knee-deep in filth that mattered, waiting for the guns to start their roaring which:

> reinforced Rivers' view that it was prolonged strain, immobility and helplessness that did the damage, and not the sudden shocks ...
> (Barker, 1992: 222)

Such a view is not confined to war, and neurasthenia, by whatever name, remains the exemplar of how illnesses can be utilised to different ends within wider contexts and situations. Money and social status can still buy you a much more user-friendly diagnosis – stress perhaps, or exhaustion – and the appropriate private surroundings from within which to recover.

Occurrences of neurasthenia had started to decrease and disappear from around the late 1920s although in parts of Asia it continues as a recognisable form of disorder, possibly because of its assumed basis in nervous system aetiology and distaste for purely psychiatric descriptions. However, around about the 1980s, there re-emerged variants of neurasthenia in the form of chronic fatigue states although lacking assumptions about an organic basis and leading some to challenge their 'real' existence as essentially neurotic in origin. What *is* clear is the cultural relevance to its different manifestations both now and in history. Its usage in World War I (this volume, Chapter 1) excused what were considered, for instance in working-class men, cases of cowardice. But there *were* no cowards, it was simply the case that social standing had a purchase on what counted as illness.

Postscript

During the Great War many officers had of course been charged with sundry offences including 'shameful conduct', 'absence' and so forth. Gerard Oram (2005) has documented these, including the full range of pardons issued to the officers by His Majesty the King, with some subsequently being reinstated and even receiving honours.

In a speech to the House of Commons (18th September 2006) Secretary of Defence Des Browne announced the government's intention to issue a group pardon to the 300 men who had been executed. In essence he said:

> The effect of the pardon will be to recognise that execution was not a fate that the individual deserved but resulted from the particular disciplines and penalties considered to be necessary at the time for the successful prosecution of the war.

The intention, he said, was to abolish the particular dishonour of execution but that the pardons did not question the procedures taken at the time which Mr Browne described as 'very difficult decisions'. In effect, the convictions remain.

References

Barker, P (1992) *Regeneration*. London: Penguin Books.

Clarke, L (1999) *Challenging Ideas in Psychiatric Nursing*. London: Routledge.

Mitchell, SW (1878) *Fat and Blood*. Philadelphia: Lippincott.

Oram, G (2005) *Death Sentences Passed by Military Courts of the British Army 1914–1924*. London: Francis Boutle Publishers.

Shorter, E (1997) *A History of Psychiatry*. Chichester: John Wiley.

DISCUSSION SIX
Chapter 9: *Macbeth*

What futures hold

Consider fate: the witches foretell Macbeth's even if they equivocate with him mischievously as though toying with his future. To what extent therefore is he responsible for his actions? He is at the mercy of supernatural forces, his future unrolling unthwarted before him unencumbered by alternatives. It's as if he's in the lap of the Gods. In Act V, sc v he senses this:

> To-morrow, and to-morrow, and to-morrow,
> Creeps in this petty pace from day to day,
> To the last syllable of recorded time;
> And all our yesterdays have lighted fools
> The way to dusty death.

That 'the fates' are in control is a view, with modifications, that does not lack historical, economic, religious and psychological support. Some of the past's most influential religious figures have preached *predestination*, a theology whose omniscient God owns the future and everyone's part in it, where salvation or damnation are already set and unalterable. Psychologically terrifying, this doom-laden scenario is not open to prayerful negotiation, indeed you can't even take it or leave it.

However, there is hope: a kind of behavioural reinforcement is at hand whereby you can assume that your work ethic, your good works generally are evidence of your being good, sufficient perhaps to be saved. From such a religiosity did philosopher Max Weber elaborate a 'protestant work ethic' which he was able to link to the expansion of capitalism. The implications are vast but, for us, it is the balm derived from how we regard our actions that matters, that we may not be predetermined, that by doing good we may persuade ourselves that we have a chance.

The alternative view is that God is sovereign but that he has given us free will, an ability to choose good from ill. However, *seeming* to possess something is not definite enough: we need to move to a more assured position than that. The problem is whether moving on represents a choice or if it's merely an inability to accept that life works its ways upon us, whether or will. So do we make the world up in some way or are we pawns in a greater and unknowable game? The essence of the debate – with many ifs and buts – is if we can exert our will on our surroundings freely or whether our lives are determined by material forces such as nervous systems.

Philosopher Mary Midgley (2001) notes that the determinists' conviction that conscious effort is futile doesn't stop them writing books about these matters, proselytising mindless determinism whilst accepting honours and rewards for *their* conscious free-willed efforts, rarely refusing the rosettes because 'life just happens anyway'. In other words, they would hardly concede that it is their neurones arriving in Stockholm to receive the Nobel, it's them.

The distinction between mind and body had been most emphatically set out by Descartes (1596–1650) to the extent that they acquired recognition as two different substances, just as Freud's later distinctions between Id and Ego would also be seen as separate entities. However it was anticipated that, at some point, mind would engulf brain, or vice versa. At the moment, the latter appears to be the case and this has significant implications for psychiatry. The heart of the problem is that insofar as brain encompasses mind, this must include consciousness and this is what has kept this question alive for four hundred years. For if true, then who (or what) is doing the believing (about things)? How does thinking affect actions – and it does – if it is part of a material realm? That would imply that it is brain activity that provides the *impression* that 'I' am 'me'. Consequently free will is a mirage, a sop to the delusion of self-determination.

Determinism in psychiatry

Behaviourists tell us that actions result from sequences of stimuli and our learned responses to them and that cognitions attending these responses are a by-product of them. Psychoanalysts, alternatively, argue that we are propelled by unconscious forces over which we, as thinking agents, have but a limited influence. The geneticists and biologists say that everything is in the blood: show me a schizophrenic and I will show you a dopamine system. In light of these, and against the wider philosophical components of the question, to what extent can anyone be said to be free and in which sense?

In April 2009, scientists reported (Leake, 2009) that they had found the neurological centre of wisdom, isolating those brain parts that become functional when humans face difficult moral problems. Professor Dilip Jeste of the University of California was reported as saying: 'Our research suggest there may be a basis in neurobiology for wisdom's most universal traits.'

By means of advanced brain scanning the research showed that the basis of this were combinations of primitive activities in the limbic system with evolved areas such as the prefrontal cortex. On the question of free will Professor Patrick Haggard of University College London stated:

Modern neuroscience is shifting towards a view of voluntary action being based on specific brain processes, rather than being a transcendental feature of human nature.

(Haggard, cited in Leake, 2009)

This is not be as stupendous as it sounds. In prosaic terms we might concede little choice over our sexual orientation or even more generally. One recalls novelist Kinglsey Amis being asked what he would have done differently in the past to which he replied: to have done things differently would have meant *being* different. So that even in the little choices we make there may be less about them that is free than we like to think and if we are merely the consequences of a past, then obviously we have little judgement about what follows. It's a dispiriting thought.

In the USA in 1994, convicted murderer Stephen Mobley appealed his death sentence on grounds of genetic deficiency submitting as mitigation his family's history of behavioural disorders. The appeal was denied on the grounds that such evidence had *not yet* reached acceptable levels of verifiability. Mobley was executed in 2005. In Britain, mental distress generally warrants leniency although the nature of the distress is central. Schizophrenia, for example, counts as mitigation because implying a belief in its physical causation, the assumption is that the person lacked rational choice. Whereas, the psychopathy of Dr Harold Shipman, who killed his patients, is not seen as mitigation since this diagnosis carries too obvious a socio-moral dimension as well as an implication of choice.

Mack the knife!

How would the Macbeths fare in the courts today? What would their claims to diminished responsibility gain them? At one point (Act III, sc iv) Macbeth cries:

I am in blood
Steeped in so far that, should I wade no more,
Returning were as tedious as go o'er.

As an aristocrat, Macbeth's lawyers would have been the best, arguing that the murders, because foretold, were out of his control, a predestination. Equally might they assert the behaviourist view that one thing just led to another, each stimulus eliciting a reluctant response and so on. Or they might assert that he was unduly influenced by Lady Macbeth – an Adam and Eve defence – that he acted under extreme duress, that she led him on.

Some resolution

Midgley (2001) says that the set of problems that sciences address have their place but that when we move towards a wider discourse we do not become redundantly subjective but, rather, that we become objective or realistic about subjectivity. Denying this is at the heart of the fate problem because it ignores that our subjectivity is always in relation to other things. If I am under attack, then I am losing certain freedoms such that I would will my situation differently. But we cannot be attacked or have our freedoms limited by our own bodies – as if they were outside events – because our bodies are ourselves. In considering fate, we have arrived at fatalism, that it matters little what we do, that our consciousness is like a stream of information inside a computer, the idiosyncratic 'us' part a mere spin-off. Macbeth the android, compelled to kill and be killed. But look again at his speech at the beginning of this discussion, the incomparable language, the uniqueness of its expression. One irretrievably opts for it as consciousness that is unique, that chooses each word with inspired delight. And even at our poor level, we must still choose fifty or more times a day, whether to go to a movie, make some toast or write a novel. Case closed. Well not entirely, because there are objective entities in the world and there are some senses in which, given how we are reared or otherwise constituted, we act in certain ways and not others. It's hard to know.

References

Midgley, M (2001) *Science and Poetry*. London: Routledge.
Leake, J (2009) Found: The brain's centre of wisdom. *The Sunday Times*, 5 April.
Shakespeare, W (1967) *Macbeth*. Harmondsworth: Penguin.

DISCUSSION SEVEN

Chapter 9: *Macbeth*

The mind–brain problem

This is one of the oldest and most perplexing questions in philosophy, the relationship between mind and brain. We can examine it by analogy to a sophisticated computer, linking its 'abilities' to its hardware and software. It has long been a fancy of science fiction aficionados that, come some glorious day, computers will independently solve problems and even attain states of feeling. Daniel Tammet (2009) recalls Alan Turing's famous test that a computer be considered intelligent if it could handle a conversation with a human. This has led to the Loebner medal being awarded annually for the programme with the best conversational ability. He says the most recent winner was 'Joan' who it seems had five million lines of conversation available to 'her'. This was how she did:

Daniel: Hi, Joan, my name is Daniel.
Joan: Hi, Daniel.
Daniel: Where are you from?
Joan: Hastings; originally.
Daniel: Oh, great! I don't live far from there.
Joan: Loughborough.
Daniel: How do you pronounce that?
Joan: Well, just right forward, S-t-i-g
Daniel: Sorry?
Joan: Do you know their origin?
Daniel: Whose origin?
Joan: I'll ask again. Do you know anything about human relationship?
Daniel: I thought we were talking about Loughborough.

And it gets worse.

In Stanley Kubrick's (1968) movie, *2001: A Space Odyssey,* a programmed computer called HAL questions the judgement of the spaceship's astronauts. As one of the astronauts attempts to de-programme HAL the latter begs him to stop, declaring that he is afraid and begging him to think about what he is doing. Is this feasible, either now or in the future, that a computer could express fear and if so would the fear be 'real'?

American philosopher John Searle thinks not and invented a test called *The Chinese Room* to prove his point. It goes like this. Imagine yourself in a room where Chinese language alphabet characters are passed through to you. You haven't a clue what they mean but you have been given a guidebook which explains what they are. So that if asked whether you understand Chinese – which you don't – with the assistance of the guidebook (i.e. computer programme) you may convincingly reply 'Yes'. What this shows is that the computer can answer questions and even win chess matches against world champions – but is not *mental*: it's not what we call mind, consciousness. However this only deals with half the problem which is that if we humans are composed of a brain – a set of hardware – then how do we think, feel, have attitudes, fall in and out of love? Is there something more to us than brain? And if so, what could it be? Many of us like the idea of mind *as well as* brain since it suggests individuality, uniqueness, and, in human psychology, 'self' concepts are never far away, usually conceptualised as the major determinant of how we interact with life.

So is the problem a question of location? It certainly is! In other words, are we a brain nestling inside a cranium or is there a mind that somehow exists independently of (or in association with) this brain? If independent, where is it?

We know where the brain is and are increasingly discovering the ways in which it works: this bears on the question of whether science will ultimately explain consciousness. As we stand, science is putting forward strong claims for some mental/behavioural events such as, for example, schizophrenia, the latter 'condition' appearing to respond positively to some drugs – which work on the brain. Other claims point to some brain abnormalities – enlarged cranial spaces – where there also appear to be positive correlations with schizophrenia. However this may be too straightforward. D.H. Lawrence once stated that water was two molecules of hydrogen and one of oxygen, plus something else, the 'something' that made water wet. And this is the problem. I feel that I am unique, that I operate consciously on the world in a way that doesn't (or shouldn't) reduce all that easily to bundles of nerve tissue.

Cartesian dualism

The philosopher Rene Descartes (1596–1650) can be viewed within a Catholic religious tradition that taught (and teaches) that we are both body and soul. In declaring 'I think therefore I am' he acknowledged science as an explanatory device but without disposing of the necessity for God. His concern nevertheless was to substitute religious faith with forms of argument, for example (a) without doubt I have a mind; (b) I can doubt I have a body; (c) as such, both of these are not identical. Another argument might be that insofar as the mind could think of things that go on for infinity, would not mind soon run out of brain which is infinite? A lot will depend on where intuition takes you: is the wetness of water its chemical structure? That the poetic and the scientific tell us about the world in different ways doesn't remove the existence of an underlying reality.

The existence of two worlds brings relief to those who would rather avoid the thought that when the brain dies so do they and this is a powerful force in humanity. Second, and of major import today, we are reluctant to allow 'I' or 'we' to boil down to an evolved collection of cells, bundles of tissue. There must surely be more to me than that? Surely I experience the world uniquely, consciously reflecting on my consciousness? But if I become depressed and am given antidepressants that make me feel better then if mind and brain are separate how come the drug works on my brain but it is my mind that got depressed?

Perhaps mind is an epiphenomenon, a secondary product of brain, a view which scientific enquiry takes as a starting point and which holds that there is an objective reality that can be made known through experiment and rational enquiry. From this perspective, mental illnesses are really brain disorders amenable to physical interventions. Professor of psychiatry Thomas Szasz has argued that since it has no observable brain pathology, schizophrenia is not an illness but rather a 'problem in living'. Of course to use the cliché: 'absence of evidence is not evidence of absence' and whilst some scientists insist that theirs is now the only way forward, others argue that consciousness is the reality that science will never touch.

Lastly, the issue of brain–mind pervades the question of free will. If what we do is a result of brain structure and how it works, where does this leave free will (or is this merely an illusion that goes unrecognised because it doesn't interfere with the general run of life)? What will happen to us when such things as mystery, doubt and love are explained?

References

Kubrick, S (1968) *2001: A Space Odyssey* [film]. Hollywood: Warner Bros.
Tammet, D (2009) *Embracing the Wide Sky*. London: Hodder and Stoughton.

DISCUSSION EIGHT

Chapter 10: *Steppenwolf*

Carl Gustaf Jung

Jung was an early follower of Sigmund Freud but he parted from him because of differences concerning the nature of the unconscious. For Jung, Freud's personal unconscious with its repressions and unresolved conflicts was unnecessarily pessimistic. In addition to being a psychiatrist, Jung had travelled very widely, including in the East, and had absorbed from other cultures their symbols and signs as well as their philosophical systems. The metaphor of the plant has been used to describe his position: the appearance of leaves and branches above ground leads to our perceiving different plants. However, these grow from a deeper, underground, a collective groundswell. So, in addition to the personal unconscious, he posited a deeper well of 'collective unconscious' where there reside archetypes of light and dark, of water, fire and other mythological entities.

Born in 1875, in Switzerland, he was convinced from childhood that he possessed a dual nature; that in addition to his everyday position in the world, he was in some way an eighteenth century adult imbued with learning, great dignity and expertise. Jung was from the first a solitary and unstable youth given to fainting when under pressure. For example, confronted with the need to learn brought considerable stress and his fainting may have helped him to avoid this. More significantly perhaps was his realisation, when he began to travel, that some of his childhood rituals involving stones and other items resembled similar practices in other cultures. It was this that attracted him to the importance of universals in language and symbols and that this might possess relevance to how the human unconscious is structured.

This brought psychoanalysis into a different sphere whilst not entirely breaking with it. Freud, with most of his acolytes, continued to address consciousness from a personal, essentially reality based, standpoint, many indeed believing that biological explanatory mechanisms would eventually emerge to back up their theories. Jung, however, took matters away from the personal, claiming a truer 'level' of consciousness, one that was transcendental in its universality and mysticism. In its application within psychiatry Jungian thinking would suggest that the cosmos forces its way into human thought in instances where, for instance, schizophrenic talk resembles, symbolically, material from ancient texts of which a patient could not have knowledge.

This is a far cry from concerns about infantile conflicts and fantasies and suggests that the issue for Jungian therapy is how to integrate parts of the person and that which collectively envelops them from timelessness and its impacting symbols. In Hesse's *Steppenwolf* we saw how mythical archetypes enter the dreams and imaginations of Harry Haller and where the goal (of the novel) is to reconnect him with his shadow, to reveal the anima to him so that he can bring it to realisation in his consciousness. Note too in *Felicia's Journey* (this volume, Chapter 8) how Ireland's history is depicted, as it so often has been by its people, as 'Mother Ireland', mother earth being another of the great Jungian mythologies and a powerful influence on people's beliefs and fears.

The dream

Freud had called the dream 'the royal road to the unconscious' with therapeutic interpretations based upon the belief that the dream's content constituted hidden wish fulfilment. That is, the actual or manifest dream had to be analysed for its real, deep-seated, relevance. Jung alternatively paid great attention to the manifest dream placing his trust in translating its symbols, seeking ways of extending these into the life of the patient. So the dream work of the analyst and patient is not about finding what grubby bits might lie underneath but is, instead, a kind of mystical journey towards an enlightened view of the self in the world.

The contrast with Freudian practice could not have been greater. The Freudian approach settled into a couch-based set pattern fairly quickly. Jung though did not prescribe any way of doing therapy since this would have contradicted his open-ended approach to exploration. But a warm relationship is established and the therapist becomes a kind of wise guru who takes his disciple along the way to truth and a higher wisdom about life. They sit opposite each other and the patient may draw pictures or engage in some sculpture. The transference (see discussion of Freud, pp. 198–201) is dispensed with, that is, it is ignored! It is as if the neurosis, whatever its nature, is less the issue than facing it calmly and intellectually working one's way towards assimilation with the wider social and philosophical sphere (see Kovel, 1978).

Unsurprisingly, it is a way of doing therapy where holistic notions of everything being connected up in history and in the here and now is an acceptable premise. Rogerians would not find it entirely alien! The approach is said to be favoured (and most suitable) for those who are perhaps advanced in years and whose sought truths may be wrapped up somewhat in the spiritual. It involves a release of imagination and an invitation to the patient to integrate not only his male/female archetypes but also the self and the infinite which are, after all, the same.

Afterword

As I mentioned in Chapter 10, you need to be careful when approaching Jungian theory and especially his teachings on imagery, symbols and the like. Farhad Dalal's (1988) paper was quite clear on the issue as are others. In particular, it would appear that Jung held anti-Semitic views and that he regarded the consciousness of the 'primitive' as less developed than that of Europeans. Neither is there anything to be gained by claiming that such views were endemic to this or that historical situation, that's no excuse. Nor do attempts to ground his racism using some of the subtleties of his writings on ancient civilisation carry water either. But that this should remove his work – whether in theory or practice – to some psychology dump is for the individual to decide.

References

Dalal, F (1988) Jung: A racist. *British Journal of Psychotherapy, 4,* 263–79.
Kovel, J (1978) *A Complete Guide to Therapy*. Harmondsworth: Penguin.

DISCUSSION NINE
Chapter 13: *The Good Soldier*

Attribution theory

'Naïve psychology', the psychology of the 'man in the street', plays an important role in human affairs both formal and informal. We size people up every day as we proceed through work and play and, even when employing formal assessment methods, intuitive assumptions play their part in interviews and other occupational appraisals. Attribution theory is formal or academic psychology's attempt to give some credibility to this, to make 'guessing psychology' more explicable in cognitive and professional terms. To that end, it can be seen as a forerunner in the developing concern of social psychologists to accord an important status to cognitive dimensions of human behaviour.

For Heider (1958), behaviour followed upon internal and/or external drivers which he called dispositional and situational attributions respectively. Most of us operate along dispositional lines: that is, we attribute intention to other people's actions, playing down or ignoring the circumstances that attend them. Therefore we attribute a loss of temper (say, in a boss) to the 'fact' of his *being* bad-tempered. So if someone asks: 'why has the boss has lost his temper?', we reply: 'because he is bad-tempered'. If, however, we are then asked: 'why is he bad-tempered?', we reply, 'because he loses his temper'. The circularity is neat (too neat in fact) but it nevertheless remains for many an attractive and effortless way of explaining human action. If we throw in the concept of 'the primacy effect' – the idea that first impressions last – then initial exposure to someone's loss of temper, despite subsequent contradictory examples, consolidates the impression that he is bad-tempered *by disposition*. Heider's theory robustly underpins much of our social lives. For instance, it solidifies male chauvinist thinking about women's behaviour such as driving, and the comedian Jim Davidson has made a career out of telling us how they can't reverse. It also drives the minds of racists and its power, made explicit by Skinner (1974), comes from the discovery that it needs but one or two incidences (or reinforcements) to confirm the mindset or stereotype.

There is, however, one instance when dispositional attribution fails and we become, instead, situational dispositionalists: any idea when or where? Why, when we consider our *own* actions, of course. In such instances we become marvellously adept at bringing into play each and every circumstance under which we must or must not act. 'What do you mean, lost my temper? So would you if you were under the kinds of pressure I am!' 'Of course, I didn't hand in my essay on time: lazy? Not me; I had to do an exam as well and, besides, my computer broke down so I couldn't print my essay out'. (Let me say as a university lecturer, that some students should be awarded rosettes for the number of times their computers fail to print out their essays on time.) We will utilise Attribution theory as we plough through *The Good Soldier*, looking especially at how people gloss over the situational factors that influence others' decisions whilst conveniently judging *their* actions and ideas as a factor of their dispositions.

Classically, in clinical psychiatry there occurs a massive attribution of disposition when we infer causal relationships between genetics, chemistry and biology and a patient's behaviour. Notwithstanding impressive studies on situational factors and depression (Brown & Harris, 1978), the predominant view still coheres around predisposition over which patients have little control. Of course it might be asked fairly if one's choice of pathology as a causal factor over and above environment is itself a free option and no doubt some groups, mental health nurses perhaps, feel trapped within settings determined by medical languages and procedures.

Predictive factors

The expectedness of a person's behaviour is a pointer towards how we assess it. We infer less about people who generally correspond to the norms of their surroundings and more about those who 'break the rules'. This is because we have more to go on in the latter cases. Consequences also tell a story. If something has many positive outcomes, for example if a play is critically acclaimed, there are packed audiences and the money is excellent, this tells us something about an actor who sticks with the role. But when the audiences are thin, the money poor but the play acclaimed, we can infer a great deal more. These are but a few of the factors that underpin attributions, and there are many others (see Horsterling, 2001).

As a theory it seems to tolerably define how we try to evaluate others and the reasons for acting as they do. Yet we must be careful, for in the detail we can still get matters wrong, particularly when we assume that others are of like mind (to us). This bias is especially telling when asked to estimate the beliefs of similar cultures to our own. In our tendency to associate with our 'own kind' we can run off in seriously wrong directions. We may be more accurate in assessing the dispositions and situations if the group is unknown to us or if we have relatively little experience of it.

Equally are we swayed by the nature of information that is fed to us. We have noted how the drama of a single lost temper grabs attention forcing a jumping to conclusions even where the evidence points another way. Personally you wouldn't be able to get me on an aeroplane for love nor money although pavements are more dangerous even when just walking on them. The invisibility of a million planes taking off and landing is overwhelmed by a single news item with its attendant photograph of the crash. Like Jim Davidson and his bad woman drivers, the evidence of one or two reinforcements is enough to blind me.

Locus of control

Julian Rotter (1966) believed that people act from either an internal or external locus of control, that some of us are able to perceive links between our actions and their likely positive outcomes, as in we have some control over events. Others – the kind likely to buy lottery tickets – see life and its chances as external attributes, things happen anyway. It's an intriguing idea although its influence has waned with critics suggesting that behavioural choices may differ according to context and particular situations. As with all attribution theories, nature versus nurture also has a place and contemporary researchers have looked at variable life patterns such as rearing habits or economic influences that bear down on decision styles. There is some evidence that training programmes can enhance internal locus of control if that is what is desired, albeit this could mean that you will never win the lottery!

With the Dowells and the Ashburnhams we can see how their backgrounds and the expectations these elicit drives them to attributions that reveal their prejudices as well as their need to construct 'society' in predictable ways. They are irreversibly content to see life in an assured, confident, style and it is only when cataclysmic events rupture this cosiness that the attributions are revealed to be as dismal as social ditchwater. Thus do attributions, made from a million standpoints, nullify any sort of external reality. In effect, we make things up as we go along.

References

Brown, GW & Harris, T (1978) *The Social Origins of Depression*. London: Tavistock.

Heider, F (1958) *The Psychology of Interpersonal Relations*. New York: John Wiley.

Horsterling, F (2001) *Attribution: An introduction to theories, research and applications*. Hove: Psychology Press.

Rotter, JB (1966) Generalised expectancies of internal versus external control of reinforcements. *Psychological Monographs 80*, 1–28.

Skinner, BF (1974) *About Behaviourism*. London: Jonathan Cape.

DISCUSSION TEN

Chapter 13: *The Good Soldier*

Projective identification

Like all of the psychoanalytic 'mental mechanisms', projective identification (PI) is argued to operate outside conscious awareness. Its theoretical gestation goes back some hundred years but for the purpose of this discussion I will attend to only one of its forms, certainly its most referenced.

The brainchild of (Austrian-born) British psychoanalyst Melanie Klein (1882–1960) PI was introduced in 1946 as a cornerstone of 'object relations theory' which pulled back the origins of neurosis from Freud's middle childhood to the weeks, even days, following birth. Sometimes referred to as 'the British School', Kleinian psychoanalysis gained favour in Britain within a pre-existent and well-established branch of paediatric medicine. PI however is now employed throughout psychoanalytic practice and has generated a huge literature since its inception.

Object relations differs from Freudian theory in that it puts less stress on instinctive drives of aggression and sexuality, instead emphasising human relationships as an important factor in development. The term 'object' is used peculiarly here insofar as it actually denotes 'subject' and the relational element is about how we begin, and continue, to relate to these objects differently. Relationships are central to the child in respect of their acquiring a confident and dependable comfort zone. This springboards into later therapeutic life where the role of the therapist becomes one of forming a safe, holding, relationship.

Essentially objects can be people or even transitional things which the child incorporates into an expanding self. We have a poor sense of identity in early life and it is contact with significant others that provide us with the rudiments of a personality. As time (and life) passes we seek those who will confirm our earlier object configurations whilst remaining blind to those who don't. There may be little enough significance in this unless, of course, earlier transitions are traumatic and so difficult to ameliorate or change in adulthood.

So the object can be conceived of as an internal representation from early relationships (usually the mother) but from others, as well, when the child begins to construct a broader social sphere. However, introjecting imagery may lead to splitting because the infant finds it difficult to hold onto such emotional traits as rage or longing. As a means of reducing their intolerableness, parts of these detested images are initially repressed but then projected outwards onto the mother. Within the first months of life the anger that baby directs at its mother's neglect (of feeding), its wrath, somehow frees it from anxiety and anger and if all proceeds reasonably well – an easy dependency evolving between them – then at about eight months the child can begin to identify both good and bad representations of objects and become reconciled to this.

However when an unsatisfied infant hurls its rage at the mother she may emit similar behaviour towards it. Unable to hold the child psychologically she too attaches blame and may, for instance, refuse to pick baby up until 'it' stops punishing her with its crying. This becomes an embryonic template from which future conflict builds; it becomes the footplate of adult neurosis. An example will explicate this. Imagine you, Helen, are walking home when you bump into Alice who says 'Gosh but you've put on weight'. You immediately feel uncomfortable. Some small talk follows after which, still flustered, you take your leave. On reaching home you find yourself looking into a mirror whilst later standing attentively on weighing scales. In fact, you haven't put on weight at all and though you suspect this you persist in the belief that you have and act accordingly. You are now the owner of ideas and feelings that have nothing to do with you. You may, if you wish, consider that Alice – has *she* put on weight or is she frightened to? – has in turn projected *her* apprehensions onto you.

Conceptually, therefore, PI is at work when an individual resolves emotional stress by falsely attributing unacceptable feelings and/or thoughts to someone else. It's not quite the same as projection because, with PI, there doesn't occur a complete disavowal of conflict be it guilt or whatever. Retaining awareness of one's misgivings, these are nevertheless misattributed to others and, as in the Helen example, this not infrequently induces projective feelings (in the other). But it is the capacity to emotionally weigh such feelings, to anticipate their resolution, that matters and this comes from one's initial internalisation of objects.

Capable of interpretation in various ways, PI is certainly a primal communication of sorts. Ogden (1979) suggests that because it creates feelings in another that are congruent with one's own it thereby induces a sense of being understood. Possibly it's a quirky ploy aimed at psychological safety. Or, it may constitute psychological cheating where assigning one's mental traumas to another involves a change of ownership, the other now having to cope with them. However the important issue is that all of this begins from birth, that elements of attachment and their disturbances take hold and having done so reverberate throughout life. So, for example, in group work, some participants intellectualise, some seek scapegoats, other's jeer, become angry or try to take over and so on. Not that that which is projected is always or necessarily negative. For instance, those with positive esteem may anticipate envy, abandonment, or jealous retaliation (from others). That being so, they may seek to discharge their better 'self' into a significant other as a deflection of danger, a kind of 'head in the sand' manoeuvre wherein the bits that annoy cannot be seen.

We must not leave professionals out of the equation. Psychoanalysts spend years in therapy so as to understand the paradoxical and conflict-ridden unconscious domains, including their own, which are at the heart of therapy. What transpires between therapist and patient is of their own making and therapeutic responses may be elicited by what patients say. Both skill and pain are operant here but insofar as matters wrestle between reality and fantasy they defy common sense or the language of the educated. If a therapist is re-created as demonic by his patient, the key to resolving this will turn on the analyst's willingness to inculcate tolerability of the unresolvable (between them both) and this requires an emotionally primitive space that only a safe boundary can provide.

The emblematic languages of post-analytic therapies are each generation's need for a newer anti-neurotic rhetoric. But the final redress in any therapy is not just the offer of containment or growth but an understanding of what psychic pain is like. PI, by any other name, exhumes truths about the futility of everyday discourse and the ubiquity of disillusionment.

It doesn't take much figuring out as to why Freudian theory lends itself to literature and the arts generally more than any other psychology. What's perhaps annoying (to professionals) is when literature does the job better as it seems to do in *The Good Soldier* where so much that happens is predicated on the psychoanalytic principle that we know much less about ourselves than we like to think.

In *The Good Soldier*, Dowell is unable to express sexuality. Though he doesn't lack emotion, his attempts to deal with this are so tinged with denial that it *invites* his wife's duplicity and whose extramarital sexuality in turn is 'justified' in her consciousness by his sexual incapacities. And at he end of the novel (p. 161) when he declares: 'I loved Edward Ashburnham ... I loved him because he was just myself', this is as clear a declaration of projective thinking as you will get, a naïve eunuch, unable to see what and who Ashburnham really is, preferring instead to see what he wants to see, and serving the purpose of sustaining an indefensible social system. And why? Because, says Dowell: 'society must go on; it must breed, like rabbits. That is what we are here for. But then, I don't like society – much' (p. 161).

He knows this is a queer situation to be in, but then how can anybody be certain of anything in affairs of the heart or mind: how can we know anything?

A word of warning

Over-determinism is the error of ignoring that there may be various and different factors to account for a phenomenon. This may matter little in therapy but when, for example, projection is used to explain racial hatred where the identified inferiority of 'the other' is the projection of my own inferiority, and where I then begin to *perceive* in the other, examples of that which is deficient, this invites trouble. There is a danger when psychology is pushed too far into the social and/or political domains especially if other factors, including moral, are not taken into account.

Reference

Klein, M (1946) *Envy and Gratitude and Other Works*. London: Hogarth Press.
Ogden, T (1979) On projective identification. *International Journal of Psychoanalysis, 60*, 357–73.

INDEX

A

Abbott, EA 11, 17
Achebe, C 162, 163, 172, 193, 194
Africa/African 19, 21, 167, 168, 170
   despots 193
   history 192
   writing/writers 161–4, 193, 202
alcohol/alcoholism 41, 46, 156, 199
allegory i, 11, 87, 180, 193
Altschul, A 149, 158
Alvarez, A 46, 54
Amis, Kingsley 11, 12, 17, 20, 25, 39, 40,
     54, 104, 176, 177, 184, 185, 207
Amis, Martin 42, 45, 54, 91
Anozie, S 162, 172
anti-psychiatry 22, 23, 80, 92, 189, 195
anti-Semitism 52, 123, 124, 214
Appignanesi, L 78, 81
archetypes 138, 139, 140, 213
Arendt, H 123, 124, 128
Armstrong, PB 177, 184
Ashcroft, B 192, 194
Attribution Theory 180, 215–16, 217
Atwood, Margaret 24, 25
Austen, Jane 9, 10, 17
autobiography 22, 40, 41, 47, 69, 139,
    159

B

Bair, D 22, 25
Baly, M 76, 77, 81
Bannister, D vii, 16, 17
Barker, Pat 38, 203, 204
Barnes, M 81

Bateson, G 81, 86, 99
Bauby, J-D i, iii
Bayley, J 117, 128
BBC News 172
Beard, George 76
Beckett, Samuel 14, 22, 42, 54, 123, 128
behaviourism 20, 48, 52, 61, 97, 117, 171,
    198, 205, 206, 207
Bennett, Alan 182, 184
Ben-Zvi, L 14, 17
Berkoff, S 98, 99
Berne, E 119, 128, 186, 187
Bhabba, H 164
black radicalism 163–4
blood 123, 125, 194
Bloom, H 88, 99, 120
Blunden, Edmund 27, 36
Boorman, J 77, 82
Borges, JL ii, iii, 185, 187
Bourne, H 79, 82
Bradbury, Malcolm 149, 158
Bradford, R 12, 17, 50, 54
Bradley, AC 122, 128
Brindley, M 169, 172
British army 101, 204
   and class 203–4
   General Routine Order 37
Bronte, Charlotte 59, 67
Brooke, Rupert 27, 31, 33, 34, 36, 38
Brown, Des 204
Brown, GW 30, 38, 130, 143, 171, 172,
    185, 187, 216, 217
Budgen, F 154, 158
Burchill, J 13, 17
Burgess, Anthony 9, 17
Burgess, Guy 182

Burleigh, N 63, 67
Burls, AP 169, 173
Byatt, AS 153, 158
Byron, Lord 19, 25, 55
'Byronic Hero' 59

C

Calder, J 90, 99
Calvinist theology 90, 136
Calvino, Italo 12, 17
Camus, Albert 185, 187
Canetti, E 185, 187
Carothers, JC 171, 173
Carruthers, G 109, 110
Cartesian dualism 210–11
Cary, Joyce vi, viii, 185, 187
catholicism 105, 125, 156, 174, 176, 178,
        210
character/s, fictional vii, 33, 36, 174, 179,
        186 (see also protagonist)
    as linguistic construction 12
    and meaning 14
    Machiavel, the 112–13
    unreliable narrator 17
    Vice, the 56, 57, 112
Charles Manson gang 123, 127
Charon, R i, iii
Chase, J 164, 173
chauvinism 24, 46, 150, 187, 215
childhood 60, 148, 198, 218
    trauma 105, 134, 142, 199
Chinese room 210
chronic fatigue syndrome (see also
        neurasthenia) 27, 76, 202, 203
Clare, Anthony 146, 189
Clark, Alan 47, 54
Clarke, L 28, 38, 80, 82, 94, 99,
        149, 158, 170, 173, 202, 204
class 24, 35, 36, 76, 130, 131, 153, 175,
        178, 182 (see also social order)
    and gender 29
    and mental illness 23
    and war (see war and class)

Clemen, W 60, 67
Clinton, Bill 63, 64
Cocteau, J 60, 67
cognitive behaviour therapy (CBT)
        15, 16, 22, 79, 97, 201
Cohen, Leonard 123, 128
colonial/ism 161, 162, 164, 193
Comfort, A 54, 89, 99
comic despair 51–2
community
    -based gardens 169–71
    for people with psychosis 91 (see also
        therapeutic community movement)
    psychiatry 86
consciousness 114, 124, 125, 131, 148,
        186, 198, 206, 208, 210, 211, 213,
        220
control, locus of 217
Cooper, D 23, 25, 86, 99, 166, 190
Cooper, Jilly 14, 18
Coursen, HR 64, 67
Craiglockhart hospital 27, 28, 32–3, 37,
        76
culture 21, 50, 101, 106, 165, 192, 212,
        216
    psychiatric 106

D

Dalal, F 214
Dale, R 153, 158
death 10, 59, 65, 83, 84, 106, 121, 122,
        132, 137, 148, 157, 170
Del Rio Alvaro, C 22, 25, 87, 90, 99, 103,
        110
delusion/al 70, 133, 168, 183, 190
    insanity 108, 135, 140, 166
    paranoid 85, 159
    and self-deception 84
denial, psychological 20, 61, 106, 107,
        117, 180
depression v, 30, 69, 130, 139, 145, 155,
        171, 172, 177, 185, 203, 216, 221
Descartes, Rene 206, 210

determinism in psychiatry 133, 206–7
diagnosis/diagnostic 69, 76, 133, 147, 151, 153, 171, 183, 190, 203, 207
discourse vii, 163, 208
displacement 21, 41, 199
Doppelgänger syndrome 71, 135, 140
Dostoevsky, F v, vii, 135, 143, 187
Downie, R 20, 25
Doyle, Roddy 104, 110
dreams/nightmares 30, 83, 84, 107, 167, 198, 213
Driver, D 163, 165, 167, 173
Dryden, John 55, 145, 158
dualism/duality 89, 90, 131, 133, 176
    Cartesian 210–11
Duguid, L 12, 18, 24, 25, 104, 110
Durante, Jimmy 112, 128
Durkheim, E 130, 143

E

Eagleton, T 13, 18, 52
Eccles, M 59, 67
ecotherapy 169, 170
Egoyan, Atom 101, 109, 110
Ellis, AE 185, 187
Ellis, Warren 99
empathy i, vii, 22, 97
English/British 101, 106, 107, 110, 194
Enoch, D 135, 143
equivocation 64, 125–7
Esterson, A 92, 99, 191
ethnicity vi, 19, 20, 21, 186
evidence 15, 37, 48
    -based practice v, 15, 16, 52, 106, 165, 172
evil 21, 56, 57, 61, 65, 66, 89, 90, 95, 101, 103, 105, 110, 112, 117, 123, 124, 140, 142, 155, 156, 171, 172
existentialism 51, 86, 87, 166, 189

F

family/ies the 10, 92, 93

and schizophrenia 80, 86, 91, 92, 133, 190, 191
Fanon, F 161, 163, 164, 167, 172, 173
Farland, M 23, 25
fascism 64, 123
Faulkes, Sebastian 37, 38, 140, 143
female/s (see also women) 40, 62
    hysteria 29, 32, 76
    sexuality 71
    and psychosis 80, 142
feminism 23, 62, 72, 167
feminist novelists 24, 75, 161
films 11, 35, 37, 56, 60, 89, 98, 109, 123, 124, 127, 142, 158, 184
Foucault, M 66, 67, 92, 187
Foudraine, Jan 183, 184
free will 48, 61, 205, 206, 211
Freud, S 28, 29, 30, 32, 38, 53, 60, 105, 119, 120, 121, 122, 123, 128, 146, 149, 198, 199, 201, 206, 212, 218
Freudian
    Macbeth 119–21
    theory 29, 30, 89, 105, 218, 220
Friedkin, W 56, 67
Fuchs, C 103, 110

G

Gaertner, J 152, 158
Gall, FJ 140
Gans, JS 87, 97, 99, 185
Garcia Márquez, G 185, 188
Garfinkel, H 20, 25, 179, 180, 183, 184
Gay, P 198, 201
gender/gendered 19, 29, 115, 117–19, 163, 166, 167, 186, 191, 199
genius 151
    /lunatic, myth of the 151–3
Gibbons, L 102, 110
Gillan, P 48
Gilman, CP 24, 25, 69, 82, 135
Goethe, JW von v
Goffman, E 24, 25, 94, 99, 119, 128, 148, 158, 179, 183, 184, 195, 196, 197

Goldberg, D vi, vii, viii, 185, 188
Golding, William 12, 18
Gopnik, A 53, 54
gothic fiction 56, 72–4, 86, 89, 148
Gramsci, A 192
Graves, Robert 28
Greenberg, M 10, 18

H

Haggard, Patrick 206, 207
Haines, F 142, 143
hallucinations 75, 135, 156, 159, 160, 168
Hammond, A 62, 67
Hardy, Thomas vi
Harrington, A 140, 143
Harris, R 14, 18
Harris, T 30, 38, 143, 171, 182, 185, 187,
        216, 217
Harris, Thomas 103, 110
Harrison, K 77, 82
Haslam, S 181, 184
Hawes, J 99
Head, Bessie 19, 20, 21, 25, 173, 192, 193,
        194
Heaney, Seamus 102, 103, 110
Heidegger, M 92
Heider, F 180, 181, 184, 215, 218
Heller, Joseph 94, 99
Henderson hospital 28, 33
Henshaw, P 52, 54
Hesse, H 9, 90, 143, 213
history 33, 80
    Irish–British 101, 103
    of psychiatry 16, 80
Hitchens, Christopher 54
Hochman, B 70, 82
Hornstein, GA 16, 18, 165, 173
Horsterling, F 216, 218
Howard, Elizabeth Jane 40, 44, 47–8, 54
Hudson, L 132, 143
Hughes, K 46, 47, 128
Hunter, GK 113, 128
Hynes, S 153, 158, 180, 184

I

identity 19
images and symbols v, 127, 138, 218
immorality 65
immortals 131, 141
infatuation 51, 139, 155
insanity v, 19, 65, 72, 108, 161, 164
insulin coma therapy 79
Ireland/Irish 102–8, 176, 194, 231
Irving, H 126, 128

J

Jacobs, E 39, 44, 52, 54
James, A 80, 82
James, Clive 124, 128
James, H 14, 18
James, Sid 127
James, W 76, 117, 128
James-Lange Theory 117
Jameson, F 193, 194
Jaspers, Karl v, viii, 190, 191
Johnson, BS 12, 18
Johnsone, N 142, 143
Johnston, I 62, 67, 117, 122, 128
Johnstone, L 81, 82
Jones, M 28, 33, 38
Jordan, Neil 104, 110
Jorgens, J 127, 128
Joyce, James 9, 18, 46, 52, 101, 154, 158
Jung, CG 105, 138, 143, 168, 173, 212
    and the collective unconscious 105,
        138, 212
    and racism 214

K

Kafka, Frans ii, 9, 10, 15, 18, 71, 99, 113,
        171, 185
Kakutani, M 148, 158
Kesey, K 20, 25
Kipling, Rudyard 130, 143
Kitchener, Lord 31

Klein, M 218, 221
Kott, J 65, 66, 67, 84, 99, 123, 128
Kovel, J 200, 201, 213, 214
Kubrick, Stanley 103, 110, 209, 211
Kuna, F 85, 99
Kurosawa, A 128, 129
Kyziridis, TC 135, 143

L

Laing, RD v, viii, 22, 23, 25, 51, 80, 83,
        86, 91, 92, 99, 129, 132, 133, 142,
        143, 148, 158, 161, 164, 166, 171,
        172, 173, 183, 189, 191, 196, 197
Lane, RJ 162, 167, 173
language v, 13, 187, 194
    perversity of 107
    psychotic 87, 161, 183
    therapeutic 29, 49, 186, 220
Lanser, SS 74, 82
Larkin, Philip 45, 52, 53
Lawrence, DH vii, 46, 210
Layard Commission 16
Layard, R 16, 18
Leader, Z 39, 45, 52, 54
Leake, J 206, 207, 208
Leff, J 92, 99, 191
Levenson, M 174, 184
Levy, Andrea 193, 194
Lewinski, Monika 63, 64
literary
    alternatives 186
    confidence trick 85
    creativity 193
    criticism 12, 46, 80
    device 20
    goalposts 141
    insights 120
    niceties 193
    tradition v, 59, 76
literature i, v, 14, 20, 75, 89, 94, 97, 135,
        159, 166, 180, 185–6, 192–3
Loncraine, R 66, 67
London, T 60, 67, 129

Losey, Joseph 35, 38
Lowman, R 146, 158
Lull, J 56, 67
lunatic 151–3, 159

M

Machiavel, the 112–13
Machiavelli, N 112, 129
MacKenna, D 102, 110
MacKenzie, C 160 ,173
MacKinnon, G 37, 38
mad/madness i, v, vii, 20–4, 71, 75, 81,
        89, 95, 122, 135, 140, 148, 150,
        152, 161–3, 167, 168, 170, 175,
        183, 185, 187, 190
Magee, B 136, 143
Maier, E 139, 143
Maithufi, S 167, 173
male malady 31
Mamoulian, R 89, 99, 142, 143
Mann, Thomas vi
Manson gang 123, 127
Mantel, Hilary 24
Mantle, J 13, 18
marriage/marital 24, 40, 45, 59, 75, 78,
        96, 159, 176–7, 183
    boredom/breakdown 142, 151, 159
    of convenience 183
    disloyalty 178
    dutiful 158
    roles 72
Maslow, AH 22, 25
McCabe, P 103, 110
McCann, C 60
McCarthy, M 20, 25
McEwan, Ian 14, 18
McGrath, Patrick 21, 22, 23, 25, 146, 147,
        158, 162
McKellen, Ian 60, 64, 66, 158
McWilliam, C 148, 158
Meixner, JA 175, 184
Melville, H 9, 18
men and war 76

mental health
  and alienation 186
  and containment 94–5
  and environment 30, 37, 38
  and gender 81
  and oppression 166–7, 192
  workers vi, 15, 16, 22, 216
mental illness v, 22, 37, 79, 80, 156,
      165, 200, 207
metaphor 119, 184
Midgley, M 16, 18, 206, 208
Millett, K 81, 82
mind–brain problem 209–10
Mitchell, S Weir 24, 72, 74, 75, 77, 78,
      80, 202, 204
Miyoshi, M 140, 144
Mobley, S 207
moral equivocation 64
morality 56–8, 65, 112, 140
Morgan, G 34, 38
Moseley, CWRD 20, 26
Muir, E 95, 99
multiple personality 121–2
  disorder 133, 134, 142 (see also
    personality disorder)
murder/er 117, 118, 121, 122, 123, 125,
    126, 127, 136, 145, 158
  and serial killers 103
Myrick, D 56, 68
myth/mythical 65, 74, 160, 165
  of the artist 46
  hero 153

N

Nabokov, V 15, 18, 83, 99
Nagel, T 84, 85, 99
narrative 9, 12, 13, 162, 174, 175
  methods 89
  of the patient 12, 16, 97
narrative/narrator 9, 11, 33, 80, 84, 93,
    113, 147, 167, 175–6, 186
  of hope 142
  methods 89

protagonist 11
structure i
traditional 12, 162, 174
uncertainty 180
Western 162
nationalism 106–7
Nazi/s 124, 136, 138, 198
neurasthenia (see also chronic fatigue
    syndrome) 27, 29, 74–7, 202–3
  treatment of 77–9
neurotic/ism 24, 54, 175, 204, 213, 218
Nichols, M 116, 129
Nietzsche, F 136, 137
Night Shyamalan, M 56, 68
Nightingale, Florence 76, 77
North, M 45, 54
Norton, RC 132, 139, 144
novels 9, 192
  post-colonial 21, 73, 101, 106, 186,
    192, 193, 194
  write-back 74, 101, 192, 193
novelists 9, 12, 22, 23, 41, 162

O

object relations theory 218
Ogden, T 219, 221
Olivier, Laurence 56, 57, 59, 66, 68,
    120
oppression 20, 155, 159, 161, 164, 166–
    7, 168
  in Africa 160
  female 81, 185
  histories of 81
  psychiatric 150
  racial 168, 193
Oram, G 204
Orley, J 171, 173
Osaki, LT 161, 173
Osborne, C 88, 99
other 167, 192
outsider 130, 132, 187
Owen, Wilfred 27, 33, 34, 36, 38
Oyebode, F vii, viii, 185, 188

P

Pacino, Al 66, 68
Padley, S 194
Pascal, R 99
Pasley, M 83, 99
passion/ate 151–2, 154–6, 174–5
Paxman, Jeremy 51, 54
Pembroke, L 80
personality disorder 101, 156, 170 (see
        also multiple personality disorder,
        and psychopathy)
person-centredness 21, 136
Petrie, D 142, 144
Pfeiffer, J 91, 93, 99
Plath, Sylvia 23, 24, 26, 46, 47
Plato 180, 184
plot, the 10–11
poetic justice 65–6
poetry 9, 13, 33, 59, 102, 103, 128, 190,
        211
    war 27, 33–4, 36
Polanski, Roman 123, 124, 127, 128, 129
political ambition 66
positivism 30, 31
postcolonial 21, 73, 101, 106, 161, 186,
        192, 193, 194, 211
    novel 102, 192
post-traumatic stress disorder 27
predictive factors 81, 216
privacy 50–1
projection 41, 51, 60, 61, 84, 110, 117,
        125, 156, 157, 199, 220
projective identification (PI) 181, 184,
        218–20, 184, 191
protagonist, the 9, 11, 17, 23, 30, 59, 65,
        114, 130, 161, 192
protestant ethic 136–7
Proyas, A 134, 143, 144
Prozac 79
psychiatric service user 37, 80
psychiatricising *Metamorphosis* 91–2
psychiatrists 22, 24, 28, 30, 36, 72, 74,
        76, 79, 91, 146, 147, 157, 189

psychiatry 16, 33, 206
    anti- 22, 23, 80, 92, 189, 195
    colonial 171–2
    determinism in 206–7
    disregard for morality 65
    Hesse and 138
    history of 16, 80
    limits of vii
    radical 23, 80, 87, 91, 92, 133, 150,
        164–6, 172
psychoanalysis 15, 20, 29, 30, 48, 49, 52,
        60, 61, 90, 140–1, 143, 150, 154,
        166, 181, 185, 191, 212, 220
    Kleinian 218
    practice of 150, 198, 200–1
psychoanalytic therapy 49, 199
psychological
    analysis 104
    anguish 85
    denial 20
    discourse vii
    distress 193
    insights 161
    knowledge vs mechanisms 180
    safety 219
    science 185
    support 205
    techniques 169
    understanding 186
psychology
    beyond 180–2
    origins of 196
psychopathy/personality disorder 21, 65,
        90, 101, 103, 156, 194, 207
    borderline 170
psychosis/psychotic 86–8, 91–3, 98, 118,
        152, 155, 162–4, 168, 171 (see also
        schizophrenia)
    and the family 91, 92, 93, 98
    and female sexuality 80, 81
    gaze 153
    speech 183
    and writing 22
psychotherapy/psychotherpist 16, 22, 45,

49, 134, 136, 165, 179, 181, 184, 185–7, 198, 200, 213, 220
Amis, K and 44–5
and class 29, 36
and medical profession 16

Q

Quawas, R 72, 76, 82

R

race/racist/ism/ial 50, 52, 53, 74, 138, 139, 159, 160–1, 186, 193, 214
and elitist medicine 164
biology of 167
bitterness 21
oppression 193
superiority 73
radical psychiatry 23, 80, 87, 91, 92, 133, 150, 164–6, 172
Ramsey, M 184
randomised controlled trial (RCT) 170
realism 11–13, 104, 131
recovery 22, 78, 97, 165, 169
and the garden 169–71
Reed, A 190, 191
repression 20, 32, 90, 110, 119, 142, 143, 183, 198
Rich, F 59, 68
Richard and Judy's book club 13
Rieger, BM 186, 188
Rivers, WHR 27ff, 203
Rogers, CR 22, 26, 113, 129, 136, 137, 144, 182
role play 58
Rosenberg, Isaac 27, 36
Rosenhan, D 23, 26
Rosenthal, D 128, 129
Rosten, Leo 39
Roth, M 73, 74, 82
Rotter, JB 217

S

Sakel, M 79, 82
Sassoon, Siegfried 27ff
and his protest 34–5
schizophrenia v, 22, 78, 80, 84, 86–7, 91–2, 96, 133, 138, 142, 149, 152, 153, 155, 160, 161, 162, 164, 189, 190, 191, 202, 207, 210, 212 (see also psychosis)
configurations of 86
existence of 189
families and 80
and first rank symptoms 187
genesis of 190
insulin coma therapy 79
radical psychiatry's view of 164
as sane reaction 189
Schorer, M 181, 184
Schreiber, FR 133, 144
Schuster, DG 77, 78, 82
Searle, J 210
Second World War 27, 33
self 66, 167
sex/sexual/ity vi, 32, 60, 61, 145–8, 151–8, 160, 178, 181, 198, 207, 218–20
aggressive 105
appetite 41
conquests 105
dalliance 147
female 71, 80
inadequate 52
licentiousness 152
myth and 168
orientation 52
and power 63
prowess 121
sadomasochistic 59, 81
status 35
undertones 143
violent 60
Shaffer, BW 21, 26
Shakespeare, W v, 13, 21, 41, 54–6, 59, 62, 66–8, 88, 92, 112, 114, 119,

120, 121, 123, 125, 128–9, 136, 152, 175, 184, 196, 197, 208
Shelley, Mary 72, 82, 144
shell shock 27, 28, 33–7
Sher, Anthony 59, 61, 68, 117, 120
Shipman, Harold 207
Shipman, T 124, 129
Shoenberg, E 90, 100
Shorter, E 79, 80, 82, 202, 204
Shotter, J 25, 26
Showalter, E 32, 38, 72, 73, 77, 78, 82
Siegel, L 60, 68
Singer, B 124, 129
Skinner, BF 132, 144, 215, 218
Smail, D 30, 38
Smiley, J 175, 184
Smith, G 59, 68
Smith, Z 193, 194
social order 21, 23, 72, 136, 175, 178, 179
(see also class)
Sorley, CH 33, 36
spiritual order 21
St Peter, C 106, 111
Stendhal vi, 185, 188
Stephen, M 34, 38
Stevenson, Robert Louis 89, 90, 100, 140, 142, 144
Stopes, Marie 71
story line 12, 13, 14, 20, 139, 140, 181, 193
storytelling 12, 14, 174, 175
suicide/alism 121, 130, 131, 157, 175
supernatural 56, 125
symbolic/symbolism 87, 128, 138, 147, 148, 212
interactionism 195
Szasz, T 23, 26, 189, 191, 196, 197, 211

T

Tammet, D 209, 211
therapeutic community movement 28, 33, 37, 79, 172
Langlan 91

Thigpen, CH 133, 144
Thirwell, A 10, 18
Thomas, P 98, 100
Thorlby, A 87, 100, 113, 129
Tóibin, Colm 176, 184
Tolstoy, L vi, 9, 10, 18, 93
Tonkin, B 148, 158
transference 78, 150, 213
Traversi, D 57, 68
Tremain, Rose 24
Trevor, Wlliam 21, 22, 23, 26, 87, 90, 101ff, 111, 194
Trotter, D 176, 184
Turgenev, I vi, 185, 188

U

unconscious 49, 61, 89, 113, 131, 132, 148, 175, 181, 182, 198, 200, 206
collective 74, 105, 138, 212
Underwood, R 77, 82
universality 74, 172
unreliable narrator 11, 17, 147, 150, 175
utopian society 21

V

Vallely, P 125, 129
Verhoeven, P 124, 129
Vice character 56, 57, 112
Vidal, Gore vi, 185, 188
von Sacher-Masoch, L 85, 100
Vonnegut, Kurt 94, 100

W

Wain, Louis 152, 153
war
and class 33, 35, 203–4
Crimean 76
impact of 17, 27ff, 37, 203
men and women and 76–7
and neuroses 30, 31, 203
trauma 28, 30, 33

Waugh, P 12, 18
Welles, Orson 127, 129
West, Nathaniel vi, viii
Westman, K 36, 38
Willbern, D 116, 129
Wilson, C 130, 131, 144
Wilson, E 96, 100
Winterson, Jeanette 24
witch(es) 114, 120, 125, 126, 205
women 40, 62 (see also females)
   in African writing 161–4, 202
   Amis, K and 40, 44–5
   inherent weakness 77
   and madness 161
   mental activity of 202
   and neurasthenia 78
   psychiatry's attitudes to 24, 25, 31, 69,
       74–5, 189
     radical 23, 24
   rights of 71–2, 75, 81
   subjection 24
   and war 76–7
   as writers 193
Woodham-Smith, C 76, 82
Wooster, G 47
write-back novels 74, 101, 192, 193
writer, the and his world 90–1
writing madness 161–3

Y

Yalom, I 132, 144
Yealland, L 30ff
Young, DAB 76, 82

Z

Ziolkowski, T 131, 144

THE HOPE OF THERAPY

PAUL GORDON

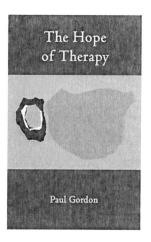

ISBN 978 1 906254 11 7
Retail Price £12.99, pp. 130

This book is an argument for therapeutic freedom at a time when hyper-regulation and state interference threaten to suffocate and dominate psychotherapeutic practice. Therapy is inherently an ethical endeavour, both in the sense that the therapist is called upon to be responsible to and for the other who seeks help, and in the sense that it is inevitably bound up with ideas about how we should live and how we should treat one another.

Therapy is not a matter of technique but is rather an art or craft and has much to learn from other forms of art and craft, such as painting, fiction, music and poetry. Like artists, therapists need to feel free if they are to be truly creative.

CONTENTS

1. The ethical space of therapy
2. The limitless conversation
3. The space of therapy
4. An aesthetics for therapy
5. A poetics for therapy
6. The hope of therapy

THE AUTHOR

Paul Gordon has been working as a psychotherapist in different settings for almost 20 years. He is a member of the Philadelphia Association and works in private practice and as a therapist to one of the Philadelphia Association community households. He lives in London with his wife and two children. He is the author of *Face to Face: Therapy as ethics* (1999) and co-editor of *Between Psychotherapy and Philosophy: Essays from the Philadelphia Association* (2004).

PCCS Books

independent publishing for
independent thinkers

www.pccs-books.co.uk